Cathy Weideman

T5-ACQ-592

Dance/Movement Therapy Abstracts: Doctoral Dissertations, Masters' Theses, and Special Projects

1991 - 1996

Volume 2

Sharon Chaiklin
Editor

Marian Chace Foundation
of The American Dance Therapy Association
Columbia, Maryland

Copyright © 1998 by the Marian Chace Foundation
All rights reserved. No form of this book may be reproduced in any form or by any means without written permission of the publisher.
Library of Congress Catalog Card Number: 92-72987
ISBN 1-881766-04-7
ISSN 1064-7538
Chaiklin, Sharon (Ed.)
Dance/Movement Therapy Abstracts: Doctoral Dissertations, Masters' Theses and Special Projects 1991 - 1996. Volume 2/Sharon Chaiklin (Ed.)

Marian Chace Foundation
of the American Dance Therapy Association
Suite 108, 2000 Century Plaza
10632 Little Patuxent Parkway
Columbia, Maryland 21044-3263

Contents

Acknowledgements .... *i*

Introduction .... *iii*

Abstracts 1

Index 117

Procedures for Obtaining Dissertaions, Theses and Special Projects 125

Form to Correct, Update or Submit Information 127

Acknowledgements

I am most grateful for the work of Anne Corraro Fisher who with Arlynne Stark created the first volume of this series. This initial work has made developing this second volume so very much easier in that there was a fine model to emulate.

The support of the other Marian Chace Foundation trustees, Ann Lohn and Jane Wilson Downes, enabled the energy to remain on task.

Concrete help was afforded by Harris Chaiklin through his knowledge of computers, Frederica W. Kuppers and Liz Hagerman in the typing and editing of abstracts on to the computer disk and Jessie Newburn who put it all in shape. Thanks for just being there for me.

Most of all, we thank the many students who put so many hours into thinking, creating and writing their ideas into a body of literature that is the source of that which sustains the profession of dance/movement therapy.

We most gratefully thank their many teachers who shared their knowledge in order that dance/movement therapy may continue the process of growth through their students.

Additionally, much appreciation is sent the directors of the dance/movement therapy programs who participated through their teaching and then sending the many abstracts of their students. You make this all possible.

Introduction

The Marian Chace Foundation remains committed to gathering, preserving and distributing the many theses, dissertations and special projects completed in dance/movement therapy. The Foundation's purpose in funding this collection is to make available the totality of the creative efforts, ideas, information, conclusions and recommendations of its students and practitioners. It is hoped that this will stimulate further research, writing, and theoretical development in the profession, so needed in substantiating the value and depth of clinical work in dance/movement therapy.

Based upon the inital work in Volume I which was a guide to that which was written through 1990, Volume II includes those theses, dissertations and special projects written between the years 1991-1996. It is planned that this will be a continual series of publications that will demonstrate the breadth and depth of the thinking being done in dance/movement therapy through the years.

The thesis abstracts were gathered from graduate dance/movement therapy programs that graduated students through the included years. There are several abstracts included that individuals wrote about dance/movement therapy who did not attend recognized programs. These were remitted to the Foundation in response to the notice in the American Dance Therapy Association newsletter. Doctoral dissertations were similarly included.

There are several theses which were omitted from Volume I inadvertently and these have been included in this volume along with a few corrections that were received. This will explain why the reader might see titles included written before 1991.

Although every attempt has been made for accuracy and completeness, this volume is sure to have omissions and errors. For these I offer my apologies and hope that the reader will provide any information that is needed to supplement future publications.

The book is organized alphabetically by authors' last name. If there is a known name change, it follows in parentheses. The title of the written work is listed, followed by the name of the academic institution, and year the work was submitted. The abstract follows; only a few were not available. Some of these have been edited for reasons of length, but the author's terminology, style and information remain true to what was received.

In order to identify doctoral dissertations, special projects and corrections, the information follows the heading making use of the identifying letters listed below:

Doctoral dissertation or doctorate (D)
Special project (SP)
Correction from Vol. 1 (C)

An Index follows the format of Volume I with additions that seem appropriate and necessary. That format was based upon headings suggested by the American Psychological Association in Thesaurus of Psychological Index Terms. These are headings commonly used in indexing and retrieving psychology-related subject matter. Many abstracts are cross-referenced by more than one subject matter.

A section called Procedures for Obtaining Dissertations, Theses and Special Projects then follows which suggests methods of obtaining the entire written work if desired.

It is hoped that this reference guide will be of use to others in their own learning and in enabling the larger professional and lay public to recognize the importance and intrinsic value of dance/movement therapy.

Sharon Chaiklin
September 1, 1998

Abrahamsen, Synnove J. *Eating Disorders: A Personal Growth Issue for Dance Therapists In Training.* Hunter College, 1992.

Students entering the field of dance therapy are predominantly women who have had dance training. As these students are a logical target for eating disorders, a questionnaire was implemented which included responses from two classes of dance therapy and dual degree students. This was to determine if there are any trends toward eating disorders and other related issues.

A background into eating disorders is given that focuses on three components: clinical definition, social aspects, and psychological development. Dance therapy is also discussed as treatment for eating disorders.

Although conclusive evidence for clinically defined eating disorders was not established, eating disorder behaviors were indicated. The most significant finding in the research was the high percentage of body size dissatisfaction among the students. Clearly, if a dance therapist is to function using her body as a tool in therapy, these issues need to be recognized if not resolved.

Abrahamson, Gail. *The Implications from Dance/Movement Therapy with Adolescent Populations.* University of California, Los Angeles, 1993. (SP)

Adams, Susan Leigh. *The Symbolic Meaning of the Circle in Relation to Healing in Dance Therapy.* Hunter College, 1996.

The circle functions as a symbolic and structural form in rituals, art, dance and healing, specifically psychotherapy and dance therapy. As an archetypal image, the circle instills a sense of wholeness and universality and the ensuing well-being that accompanies the feelings of belonging to something greater than ourselves. In this sense circle has significance in the healing of the individual and the community. To prove this premise, examples are provided regarding how the circle has been utilized in healing rites as well as in current psychotherapeutic practices (such as in group process, archetypal psychology and dance therapy). This thesis attempts to illustrate how the circle in ritual has curative effects. Primary in its therapeutic value is that it gives meaning to one's life through the continuous connection with others.

Dance alone has great curative potential. As a kinesthetic process it connects one to their emotions and allows cathartic discharge of emotion. One also shares this experience with others in the circle of dance, inducing a feeling of acceptance and commonality with others. Humans have an inherent need for symbolic experience. Dance therapy obtains great potential for healing due to its utilization of two proven curative means; the circle and the dance. These two elements provide the context for the process of dance therapy which can be akin to ritual, which is also proven to have curative potential.

Adderley, Michael. *The Healing Effects of Junkanoo Dance in the Bahamas and Its Relationship to Dance Therapy.* Hunter College, 1996.

This thesis examines dance and dance therapy, and in particular, the history and healing effects of Junkanoo dance in the Bahamas. Comparisons are drawn between Junkanoo and dance therapy, as it relates to the positive effects that Junkanoo continues to have on the individual Bahamian, as well as the entire country. This theory is based on the fact that the people of the Bahamas have been enjoying this grand event for many decades, which the author feels can easily be referred to as "dance therapy".

Ahroni (Barkai), Yael. *Analytical Study of the Anatomical Notation System.* University of Wisconsin, 1968.

The purpose of the study was two-fold 1) to reveal and explain the space-time aspects of the Anatomical Notation Sytem and 2) to present evidence of the refinement of the symbols in the notation. In the Anatomical Notation System, there are eight symbols which provide reference points for information of plane, degree of flexion, degree of rotation, general orientation of the body indicating base of support, contact point outside the body, and body contact to other body parts. Time conditions are identified.

This system was found to be compact and the immediate information provided an accurate means of recording movement. It was hoped that the information could be used as an initial step toward development of a universal movement notation system.

Alexander, Paulette. *Generating the Spirit: The Transformation of Traditional West African Dance to African American Social Dance Forms and its Implication and Meaning in Dance Therapy.* New York University, 1995.

African American social dance and its meaning and implications in dance therapy are examined. The origins of dance and its function in traditional African society is looked at to establish a link between the two dance forms. Dance in Africa is a total art which combines music, dance, voice, and verse. Dance is acknowledged in African society to possess healing qualities. It was during the middle passage that West African dance began the process of transformation. An overview of the function of dance during slavery illustrated that its meaning and purpose fundamentally remains West African in origin, yet reflects a distinct African American character. Two journal process notes are reviewed to examine transitional moments within the dance therapy session which supported social dance expressions of the clients.

Anderson, Kathleen R. *You are Not Alone: The Use of Dance Movement Therapy With Geriatrics.* Antioch/New England Graduate School, 1992.

This thesis examines the process by which reality orientation is stimulated within the dance movement therapy group which serves the elderly in different stages of dementia. The difficulties that occur due to the nature of this population are outlined. The essential elements which assist in creating, and maintaining attention within the group are discussed as part of the literature review. Through a clinical case study, examples of heightened awareness and reality orientation in the elderly that occur within the dance therapy session and some of the stimulators of this phenomena are demonstrated. One video taped session of the authors' dance therapy group is analyzed by Virginia Eicher, a student of Sandel's, according to Sandel and Johnson's Structural Analysis for Movement Sessions to present an evaluation of what interventions may assist the therapist in maintaining reality orientation with this geriatric population. Suggestions for future research are made. Conclusions about dance therapy as an effective form of achieving cognitive stability in geriatric clients are presented.

Angeloro, Valerie M. *Sharing The Lead: A Study of the Evolution of an Authentic Movement Group From Single Leadership to Shared Leadership.* Antioch/New England Graduate School, 1992.

This is a case study of an Authentic Movement group's transition from single leadership to shared leadership. The five group members were interviewed at the beginning of their transitional process. Interviewing was repeated six months later. This paper examines how the group members made this transition. Through insightful and responsive leadership the group was prepared for taking on the responsibility of shared leadership. After the members make a commitment to each other to continue the group, they consciciously defined the essential characteristics of their new structure. Commitment to one another and the Authentic Movement form supported shared leadership. Member empowerment resulted from this interdependent model. Empowerment further increased the members' commitment to the group and encouraged interdependence and sharing. Application of Authentic Movement to professional peer development is discussed.

Angert, Gwen. Correlating Physical Strength with Body Esteem in a Female Osteoarthritic Population. Allegheny University of the Health Sciences (formerly Hahnemann University) 1994.

There has been much study on the relationships between physical activity, aging, and psychological well being. One aspect of physical activity, muscular strength, and one psychological construct, "body esteem" are examined using thirty, 50 to 80 year old female osteoarthritic patients at the Hahnemann University Arthritis Clinic. A Body Esteem Scale (Franzoi and Shields, 1984) is administered and a Muscle Manual Test (Daniels and Worthingham, 1980) is also administered for determining the physical strength ability of this population. This researcher's hypothesis is that osteoarthritic women with low physical strength would have lowered body esteem scores, and osteoarthritic women with higher physical strength scores would have higher body esteem scores. A woman who scores high is in the domains of how satisfied she feels in the area of her sexual attractiveness, weight, and overall physical condition. A person correlation of specific and total body esteem with total strength ability is computed. Results from this study indicate no correlations between body esteem and physical strength dimensions. A discussion of the nature of the osteoarthritic female population and the limitations of the measurement tools utilized are explored, and suggestions are given for future areas of research.

Arakawa, Kayoko. *The Structure of the Japanese Sense of Harmony and the Obsessive-Compulsive Personality in Dance-Movement Therapy.* Naropa Institute, 1991.

The primary hypothesis of this study is that the experience of dance movement provides an excellent therapeutic tool of psychotherapy—especially for helping Japanese people when they are confronted with a foreign cultural and social environment.

This study will examine aspects of Japanese behavior in a different sociocultural context. It is important to recognize social and cultural patterns of behavior in order to understand problems in therapeutic techniques, both in individual or group psychotherapy. The author examines the sense of harmony within the Japanese, and how this sense is related to the sense of shame and guilt.

Also addressed is the obsessive-compulsive personality. Maintaining social harmony requires voluntary self-control rather than self-expression; therefore, function of self-control may be expected among the members of the otherwise harmonious group. Study of the obsessive-compulsive character explores what is of value and how it relates to behavior.

A case study of the obsessive-compulsive personality will be addressed in the interplay of the individual's behavior and their cultural surroundings and also discuss how culture and society interact with groups and individuals.

The thesis will identify non-verbal expressions of the character and the function of the obsessive-compulsive personality in the interaction between culture and behavior. In addition, it identifies how dance-movement therapy can benefit the Japanese patient.

Arcuri, Cara Bulson. *The Effects of Individual Dance Movement Therapy on Group Interaction: A Case Study.* Antioch/New England Graduate School, 1994.

This case study evaluates the effectiveness of individual dance movement therapy as a means of influencing a child's behavior in a group environment. He was initially quiet and withdrawn, and his movements appeared rigid and narrow. It was hoped that treatment would result in increased openness, confidence, and sociability. Behavioral changes were assessed by the author and classroom staff through general observations and the Kestenberg Movement Profile. A before-treatment and after-treatment comparison was made. After 20 weeks, the subject's level of confidence increased notably. He also engaged in peer-oriented play more frequently.

Arndt, Cheryl. *Accessing Personal Truth: Process-Oriented Dance Movement Therapy.* Antioch/New England Graduate School, 1990.

Dance/movement therapy is a diverse field which has practitioners who vary widely in their approaches toward and their rationales behind their work. This paper focuses on the theories and practitioners in the field who work from a process-oriented perspective. The process-oriented perspective is explained and is seen as different from the more traditional, medical model approaches to therapy. Theories and case examples from several process-oriented dance/movement therapists are reviewed. Where applicable, the work of others outside the field of dance/movement therapy is reviewed. The conclusions drawn from this research include the suggestion that the definition of dance/movement therapy be broadened.

Arner, Julie. *A Comparative Study of the Hunter College Dance/Movement Therapy Masters Program and an Encounter Group.* Hunter College, 1991.

This thesis examines the history, process and outcome of encounter groups and related laboratory training programs. Included in the literature review is a summary of the experiential courses in the Hunter College Dance/Movement Therapy Masters Program with an outline of their goals and requirements.

A qualitative analysis was performed on the results of a questionnaire distributed to eleven students near the completion of their training in Dance/Movement Therapy at Hunter College. The results show a significant similarity between the outcomes of the participants' experience in encounter groups and the outcomes of experiences for the dance therapy students involved in the study. Comparisons are also drawn between the nature of specific courses in the program and the encounter group.

Arning, Judith A. *Dance/Movement Therapy with Multiple Personality Disorder (MPD) Patients.* Goucher College, 1992.

The purpose of this study is to investigate the specific goals, therapeutic roles, methods and techniques used in dance/movement therapy with this population through a literature review and interviews. The literature suggests the common etiology of MPD is repeated severe abuse or trauma in early childhood and is considered a dissociative disorder characterized by formation of different identities as a means of coping. Interviews with six dance/movement therapists experienced in working with multiple personality disorder patients are summarized in three categories: background, theoretical and clinical.

Results indicate that dance/movement therapists can come from a variety of backgrounds and clinical experiences and still work effectively with MPD patients. Different theoretical approaches can be used but flexibility among theoretical approaches is key. Short-term goals tend to focus around trust and safety in the environment and in themselves. Long-term goals included developing affective awareness, developing stronger awarenesss of the different personality states and integration of these. Methods and techniques include: beginning in a circle, warm up, patients chose music, relaxation techniques, encouraging leadership, mirroring others, use of transitional objects, clear boundaries set and processing of information verbally.

Ashley, Jacquelyne S. *Moving Upon the Earth: A Synthesis of Dance/Movement Therapy and Deep Ecology.* Naropa Institute, ____.

Interest in this topic has come from the study and experience of non-western cultures as an undergraduate in anthropology, personal experience as a dancer/performer, training and practice of dance/movement therapy, and time and experiences spent with nature.

The author's study of primal cultures as an anthropologist led to an interest and focus of study upon the unified expression of the arts (visual, music, dance and poetry), healing and spirituality. These elements of focus, study or experience as they are viewed in contemporary Western culture, were not separate entities. They were and still are in some cultures, a unified expression of the culture's vitality and a vehicle for healing, both of the individual, the community and the earth.

Atley, Suzanne Hastie. *In Search of a Standard Form of Assessment: The Kestenberg Movement Profile as Diagnostic Tool and Treatment Guide Integrated into The Practice of Dance Therapy.* Antioch/New England Graduate School, 1991.

The lack of a standard form of assessment in dance therapy weakens work with clients as well as communication within and outside the field. In this thesis, the use of the Kestenberg Movement Profile (KMP) as a standard form of assessment is promoted. Through presentation and examination of the KMP in general, clinical material, and an accompanying KMP, this author describes and illustrates how the KMP can be integrated into the practice of dance therapy and how it can facilitate the diagnostic and treatment process. Two notators gathered and processed the data for the clinical material section, and a mean-generated profile was constructed by averaging their results. Statistical analysis on the inter-rater reliability between notators was done using the Pearson r. It is hoped that the reader will see the tremendous clarity, depth, and richness the KMP has to offer dance therapists in their work.

Audette, Catherine. *Ecoembodiment: Embodying This Planet With Our Respect.* Antioch/New England Graduate School, 1991.

Dance/movement therapy is presented as the primary clinical treatment modality for Adolescent Conduct Disorder. Leading to this postulation is background information concerning the evolution in parental and social attitude relating to adolescence, the understanding of normal adolescent developmental stage, and the information on the etiology, diagnosis and treatment issues of Adolescent Conduct Disorder. Also discussed are the deficits in the existing treatment systems and a comparison between conventional therapy approach and dance/movement therapy. This comparison illuminates the essential employment of dance/movement therapy for treatment of Conduct Disorder.

The three major treatment issues discussed are affect/behavior modulation, interaction/socialization, and developmental tasks for the formation of age-appropriate ego-self as well as sexual identity. These treatment issues and goals are discussed with reference to main-stream psychotherapy rationale and to dance therapy clinical grounding. Recommendations are appended for the differentiation and integration of role images as a Dance Psychotherapist for effective intervention with adolescents having Conduct Disorder.

Azizollahoff, J. *Dance Therapy and Autism: A Case Study of Miss S.* Hunter College, 1992.

    The author presents an in-depth study of the evolving therapeutic relationship between herself and an autistic, mentally retarded child. The study is a detailed exploration of various treatment methods in working with the autistic child, with emphasis on dance therapy methods. Comparisons between psychoeducational treatment interventions are made which illuminates the importance and efficacy of dance therapy's union with autism.

Baker, Marcia Franz. *The Role of Verbalization in Dance/Movement Therapy with Emotionally Disturbed Children.* Goucher College, 1992.

    This study of the role of verbalization with emotionally disturbed children consists of a literature review and the analysis of videotapes. The developmental aspects of childhood, emotionally disturbed children, verbalizaton in psychotherapy with children and how it related to dance/movement therapy were all reviewed. Two female dance/movement therapists submitted four tapes each of their sessions with emotionally disturbed children. Based upon the writings of Frost (1978) and Johnson, Rasbury and Siegel (1986), the frequency of fourteen verbal categories were calculated. These included: approvals, attention, statements, clarifications/observations, comments, confrontations, directive statements, exclamations, images, interpretations, names, numbers, prods/questions, reflective statements and sounds.

    Results indicate that the verbal categories of comments, directive statements, exclamations, and prods/questions were used most frequently, averaging nine to thirty percent per session. Therapists commented that these were used to support the therapeutic process. It was concluded that verbalizations were used frequently by the subjects and that the timing of the verbalizations was important in supporting therapeutic process.

Balish-LaSaine, Denny. *Healing Through Connection: A Relational Approach to Dance/Movement Therapy with Women Hospitalized for Depression.* Columbia College Chicago, 1995.

    This study presents a new perspective on women's psychological development as a means to more accurately address the relational needs of women participating in the dance/movement therapy process. It is not an exhaustive study but rather an overview of a paradigm shift that presents a new way of thinking about the therapeutic process with women. Due to temporal constraints, the paper focuses on women's psychological growth only and does not attempt to apply this relational theory to men.

    The authors of the "Self-In-Relation" model feel that the fundamental principles underlying this theory apply to all women but acknowledge that racial and cultural differences do exist. While acknowledging the existence of different theoretical orientations, Chace's model of dance/movement therapy is the foundation for the exploration of the dance/movement therapeutic process as Chace's contributions form the bedrock of our understanding of this unique form of healing.

Bartko, Diane Patricia. *Dance/Movement Psychotherapy with Multiple PersonalityDisorder Clients.* Naropa Institute, 1992.

    Individual and group dance/movement therapy with multiple personality disorder (MPD) clients is an essential component in the treatment process. The four focuses of treatment discussed in this thesis encompass the following crucial treatment factors necessary in the treatment of MPD: MPD clients need to feel they are believed, they need creative and non-verbal modes of expression and they need to re-own their bodies. The first section is a general overview of traditional and dance/movement therapy MPD treatment approaches. It is followed by a discussion of the four focus treatment theory. A compilation and summary of the questionnaire responses is presented. A case presentation that highlights the application of the four focus treatment theory follows and the last section offers suggestions for further research. The appendices include the descriptive study paperwork, and transcripts from the case presentation.

Basinger, Maia. *Burnout, Codependency and Disease: Healing Through Dance/Movement Therapy.* Naropa Institute, 1991

Burnout can be more effectively treated if it is considered a symptom of the deeper underlying addictive disease process of codependency and that treatment results will be more thorough if the physical body is integrated with emotional, mental, creative and spiritual changes using dance therapy. The literature review uses the illness cycle as a context to present characteristics of codependency as they correlate to those of burnout, showing the developmental progression of these problems. The deeper roots of burnout and codependency in our family history, culture and individual psychological makeup are explored. Dance/movement therapy is presented and it is shown how these traits are carried in the body. Theories on recovery within the context of the healing cycle are discussed.

Bauer, Sara. *Dance/Movement Therapy in the Treatment of Adults with Eating Disorders.* University of California, Los Angeles, 1993.(SP)

Becker, Margaret G. *A Discussion of Metaphor as a Vehicle for Understanding Body Image in Dance/Movement.* Allegheny University of the Health Sciences (formerly Hahnemann University), 1993.

This thesis presents a genesis of the combination of two complex theoretical constructs: metaphor and body image. The implications of this partnership are discussed, particularly relative to the field of dance/ movement therapy. The literature reviews neurological and psychological variables of body image which supports its elusive yet principal role in personality as a whole. The function of body image in dance/movement therapy is discussed as a nonverbal phenomenon. Research concerning metaphor is presented with regard to psychotherapy in general and dance/movement therapy in particular. The spatial and gravitational elements which determine metaphor-meaning are outlined. A synthesis of the presented material supports the therapeutic value of combining the constructs of metaphor and body image. Four results of such a combination are outlined. An attempt to define acollection of units of imagery in Dance/Movement therapy is made according to their therapeutic value. Future development of an assessment tool using body metaphor is suggested.

Ben-Ami, Ruth. *An Exploratory Study Examining the Relationship Between Voice & Movement.* Hunter College, 1992.

This pilot study aims at exploring the similarities between the movement and speech patterns of people. The literature includes many research reports dealing with the two channels of non-verbal communication studies which attempt to find a correlation between personality and vocal cues. Since no studies were found in the literature dealing directly with the relationship between movement pattern and voice cues, a detailed survey was made of the research by Ekman, Friesen & Scherer (1972), which is concerned with a related subject: an attempt to find a correlation between hand movement and voice pitch.

The assumption underlying the present study is that an individual's body movement and vocal cues present similar patterns. Ten dance therapy students, all female, took part in the study. For each one of them a movement portion was recorded on videotape and a speech portion was recorded (voice) on audiotape.

Ben-Dor, Keren. *The Use of Music and Dance Movement Therapy.* Laban Centre for Movement and Dance, 1995.

Ben-Moshe, Alon. *Butoh-Therapy: Building a New Therapy Modality.* Lesley College Graduate School of Arts and Social Sciences, 1991.

The Butoh Japanese dance is a new form of dance which evolved in Japan in the nineteen-sixties of this century, and it is experienced and danced today all over the world. The purpose of this thesis is to synthesize butoh and the expressive arts into a new structure. This thesis examines the development of butoh, it's artistic resources, it's dynamics and aesthetics, and the theoretical concepts which are its core.

The thesis leads the reader to the expressive therapy field, points out its historical development, its theoretical perception, and its applications. It concentrates on the drama and dance-movement therapy modalities as Butoh contains these two forms of expression. A synthesis of the two fields, the artistic field of Butoh and the therapeutic field of expressive therapy, are developed in order to offer a new form of therapy. This new form is called Butoh- Therapy. This thesis will build the structure of the Butoh-Therapy and examine the therapeutic process. Three concrete sessions in Butoh-Therapy are given and suggestions for relevant settings for its use.

Bennett, Elizabeth. *Contraindication in the Use of Dance/Movement Therapy.* Antioch/New England Graduate School, 1996.

As in any effective treatment modality, dance/movement therapy at times yields negative results and possible contraindications. This thesis explores possible contraindications in the use of dance/movement therapy in various settings such inpatient psychiatric hospitals, outpatient treatment centers, schools, rehabilitation hospitals, nursing homes, and private practices. Five common themes evolved from the interviews with nine dance/movement therapists and one music therapist working in various treatment settings, regarding when it is advisable to use dance/movement therapy as a form of treatment. These five common contraindications include: specific populations, instances in treatment when dance/movement therapists do not use movement interventions, effects of defense mechanisms, the use of other creative arts therapies, and the client's inability to distance from the modality/art form. The findings in the five categories are compared to previous research and conclusions are drawn in reference to the importance of the findings. Reasons for further exploration of these contraindications are discussed in conjunction with the current and future role dance/movement therapy plays in the mental health field.

Benvenuto, Juliet. *Reclaiming What was Buried, Power to the People: Dance/Movement Therapy with the Apache.* Columbia College, Chicago, _____.

This thesis explores the use of dance movement therapy as a therapeutic intervention with the San Carlos Apache Indian Tribe. It documents my understanding of Apache history and culture as well as the relationships developed with the Apache during dance movement therapy sessions together.

The specific goal of this thesis is to provide information vital to future dance movement therapists working with the Apache. Its larger goal is to benefit those who work with Native American Indian groups in general. Finally, hopefully this thesis will develop empathy for the Apache by telling the Apache story, erasing some of the myths surrounding Apache culture and shedding light on the realities of modern reservation life.

The Apache identify with being part of the "Apache People" and are clear that in order to understand the Apache now, one must know where the Apache have been—as a people. Therefore although this theses uses a "case study" format, it describes a cultural history rather than individual; it examines presenting issues for the Apache as a whole and interventions are geared towards the Apache in general rather than for just one person. There is an attempt to understand the Apache from the vantage point of dominant culture as well: namely that of a professional dance movement therapist. It makes a contemporary analysis presenting psycho-social issues facing the Apache people and explores possible therapeutic interventions using dance movement therapy. Dance movement therapy is not only presented as a powerful healing modality but is also shown as a possible link between dominant and traditional cultures as a source for healing and uniting both worlds.

Berger, Kimberly. *Language of Motion: An Introduction to The Kestenberg Movement Profile.* Antioch/New England Graduate School, 1994.

Finding a language for movement has been a concern of dance movement therapists since the origins of the field of dance/movement therapy. Dr. Judith Kestenberg has given the movement observer a language to discuss these observations, complete with psychological interpretations. This system, known as the Kestenberg Movement Profile (KMP), can be a great asset to the dance therapist trained in the specifics of this profile. However, educational resources for learning this profile are currently limited. This video is designed with the intention of being a learning tool for the Kestenberg Movement Profile. It may be used by individuals trained in the profile wishing to expand their knowledge and enhance their learning. It may also be used as a teacher's aide in the classroom setting. The video documents movement elements visually. Although nothing can replace the experience of the body's learning the movement elements of the profile, this can help the student familiarize him/herself with the KMPs movement elements visually and then practice exploring these movement qualifies.

The video provides a verbal explanation and visual representation for eight sections of the Kestenberg Movement Profile (KMP): tension-flow rhythms, tension-flow attributes, pre-efforts, efforts, bipolar shaping, unipolar shaping, shaping in directions, and shaping in planes. The written portion of the thesis provides further discussion of each section of the profile and its psycho-emotional interpretation as it relates to the field of dance movement therapy. Examples of possible therapeutic applications of the profile are provided and there is a discussion of the KMP's usefulness to the field of dance movement therapy.

Berger, Miriam Roskin. *The Use of Dance As a Therapy for Personality Disturbances.* Bard College, 1956 (SP)

A rationale for the use of dance as therapy, based on physiological, psychological and social sources; and an examination of the operative processes of dance therapy. Bodily experience and expression of emotion is discussed, with focus on the philosophical views of the mind-body connection, physiology and theories of emotion, muscle tension and relaxation, kinesthesis, expressive movement, and the body-image concept. Aspects of dance expression are explored as the roots of dance as therapy. A survey of dance therapy research is presented, which encompasses the literature until 1956: fourteen papers. There is extensive description, from observation , of the work of Marian Chace, and an analysis of her theories and methods. The concept of kinesthetic empathy is set forth for the first time in dance therapy literature. A theoretical model is given, and detailed suggestions for further research.

Berman, Jane. *The Use of Energy among Experienced Dance/Movement Therapy Practitioners.* University of California, Los Angeles, 1994.(SP)

Bertz, Jill Maria. *A Developmental Comparison of Body Movement and Mental Age in Children with Down Syndrome.* Allegheny University of the Health Sciences (formerly Hahnemann University), 1995.

This comparison of body movement and mental age in children with Down Syndrome hypothesizes that the functional development level of the children as determined in movement assessment will not reflect his/her chronological age. The age of the child as seen through developmental body movement is compared to the mental and chronological ages of the child in order to establish a correlation between developmental body movement and mental age as opposed to chronological age. Two raters rated five minutes of videotape for each subject. The dependent measures were body shaping qualities, directionality and the use of shaping in planes. Mental age was established by the use of the Hawaii Early Learning Profile. The findings of this study lend support to the hypothesis. In every case, the movement age of the child was closer to the mental age than to the chronological age of the child. This finding even pertains to two cases in which the differences between movement and mental ages was the most pronounced.

Betjemann, Theodora. *Martha and Me—A Dance Therapy Perspective: A Case Study of a 36-Year-Old Female Diagnosed With Chronic Schizophrenia Paranoid Type.* New York University, 1994.

A case study in which the effectiveness of dance/movement therapy is explored in formulating an approach to working one-to-one and in a small group with a 36-year-old woman diagnosed with chronic paranoid schizophrenia. The etiology, symptoms and chronicity of the illness are examined in order to shed light on the internal experience and symptomatic behavior of the subject of this study, as well as to explore realistic goals and outcomes for her. Examples of specific therapeutic techniques are demonstrated as being effective in helping Martha relate to others. Additionally, rhythmic synchronicity and mirroring are examined as connectors as well as sometimes obstacles in helping her move toward greater self differentiation. Concrete boundary-making and limit-setting at mundane levels of movement are noted to be essential preliminary ingredients because of their symbolic implications in helping a talented, but symbiotically-regressed female begin to individuate. Impact of interventions are noted for their effectiveness outside of the sessions as well.

Binette Louise. *KMP Analysis of Moshing: The Study of a Communal Ritual Dance Among Adolescent Males of the 1990s.* Antioch/New England Graduate School, 1994.

This thesis offers an observational study of moshing. Moshing is a dance form of the 1990s, prevalent amongst adolescent males in the transitional phase of entering adulthood. Information collected on moshing, through magazine and newspaper articles, interviews, and video tape, are related to anthropological studies of ritual dances and Jungian writings on self-created rites of passage amongst adolescents in our culture. A segment of a video tape of moshing will be analyzed using the following categories in the Kestenberg Movement Profile (KMP): tension flow rhythms, efforts, shaping in directions, and shaping in planes. Information gathered from the KMP analysis and the readings are integrated and dance/movement therapy interventions for the male adolescent population under study are proposed. In conclusion, the importance of dance movement therapists studying communal activities and dances are discussed.

Blaha, Jane. *Potential Benefits of Using the Medium of Water as Potential Adjunct in Dance/Movement Therapy Work with Schizophrenic Patients.* University of California, Los Angeles, 1996. (SP)

Blatz, Amy. *Dance Therapy and the Self-Concept in Adults with Mild Mental Retardation: A Literature Review and Proposed Model.* Hunter College, 1993.
   This paper advocates techniques for utilizing dance therapy with adults with mild mental retardation enabling them to develop and maintain a positive self-concept. A review of etiological factors, the development of the self-concept, psychotherapeutic techniques used with clients with mild mental retardation and dance therapy is presented. The basic premise is that all persons with mental retardation confront powerful stigmatizing behavior. The literature attests that they are fully aware of how they are viewed and treated and able to identify feelings of low self-concept. Dance therapy is introduced as a way to gain a capacity to express feelings, reduce isolation and improve body image, consequently improving self-concept. The model presented provides concrete activities for redefining self including: body here-and-now approach, reality testing, cohesion, symbolism and use of weight. It is maintained by the author that the mentally retarded label can be accepted if clients redefine that label. This can be achieved through redefinition of the self.

Bond, Karen E. *Dance For Children with Dual Sensory Impairments.* La Trobe University, Bundoora, Victoria, Australia, 1992. (Doctorate).
   This observational study evaluates the influence of group dance therapy on social and task engagement. Dance is examined as a therapeutic mode of learning for six non-verbal vhildren with dual sensory impairments. The research strategy combined aspects of traditional empirical design with participant observation and progressive theorizing. Within this design, a two-group experiment was conducted in which an intensive dance program was compared with another innovative treatment based on play. Repeated video recordings were taken of children and then time-sampled by independent observers to assess the relative influence of Dance and Play on selected measures of behavioural engagement. To enhance the validity of observations, relevant instrumentation was designed.
   Numerical analysis constitutes one aspect of this inquiry which draws also on audio-taped field observations, anecdotal records, school reports and interviews. Qualitative procedures were adopted to illuminate patterns of engagement uncovered through quantitative measurement. Results of the research clearly show that Dance was an effective mode of expression, communication and learning for the six children within their residential educational setting. A key finding is that personal style was an important mediator of child engagement in Dance. This finding provided a framework for three case profiles which highlight differences and similarities in personal style. In addition, the study suggested that personal style was a reflection of asethetic perception.
   In conclusion, a high level of social and task engagement in Dance appeared to be associated with an accommodation of personal style. Simultaneous consideration of the findings as they related to Dance content and methods illuminated a group process, referred to as 'aesthetic community'. A feature of aesthetic community was the emergence of a collective style of movement that encompassed both children and adults in Dance. Finally, a synthesis of research data, theory and the researcher's interpretations culminates in "Right Dance", a prototype of group dance for nonverbal children with dual sensory impairments.

Boone, Elizabeth A. *The Use of Creative Arts Therapies on a Geriatric Medical Psychiatry Unit in the Treatment of Alzheimer's Disease.* Antioch/New England Graduate School, 1996.

Dementia in the form of Alzheimer's disease is one of the most prevalent forms of psychiatric illness in the country, effecting more that 4% of those over 65 years old (DSM IV). The creative arts therapies have been developing in this country over the past 50 years and are becoming a valuable form of treatment for various populations, including Alzheimer's disease victims. The Clinton Hospital Geriatric Medical Psychiatry Unit in Clinton, Massachusetts is a short term, acute care facility specifically designed for geriatrics. This hospital is an excellent example of the incorporation of a creative arts therapy program into a treatment plan for Alzheimer's disease patients with exacerbated symptoms. A thorough exploration of the benefits of this integrated program draws from experience during a six month dance/movement therapy internship.

Booth, Heather. *Adolescent Bereavement and The Creative Process with an Emphasis on Dance Movement Therapy.* Antioch/New England Graduate School, 1995.

Adolescent bereavement is an area that has been overlooked in the past. Not much has been written on this subject, resulting in a lack of academic literature. The same is true of expressive therapies. The purpose of this paper is to examine why adolescents have a difficult time dealing with a death in the family or that of a friend. Why is loss through death different from other losses teenagers experience, such as divorce, friendships, childhood, or moving to a new locale?

This thesis explores whether adolescents can express their grief better on a nonverbal level especially through movement and other expressive arts therapies. The author wants to research, how a person experiences the bereaved body as it pertains to the following questions: What happens to the postural position of the body? How does the individual move normally and how does that differ after a death in the family? How does one examine the emotional impact and the psychological development of grieving teenagers?

Borenstein-Saks, Michal. *A Content Analysis of a Therapist's and Clients' Verbalization: A Comparison Study Between Two Dance Therapy Groups.* Hunter College, 1982.

This study is aimed at better understanding verbal phenomena in dance therapy. Attention is placed on the communication between therapist and patient, particularly its verbal expression. In order to study the verbal communication in dance therapy, two groups, led by the researcher, were tape recorded. The groups differed one from the other by the setting, the age of the patients, and by the type of population. After transcribing the tapes of the two sessions, a content analysis was conducted, and categories of verbalization were developed. A comparison between the results of the two groups has been made. The analysis showed a difference in both groups with regard to the leader's verbal behavior as well as the client's verbal behavior.

Boyle, Brian. *Male Dance/Movement Therapists.* Hunter College, 1992.

This study describes the reasons why there are so few males in the field of dance/movement therapy and examines the experience of males who do enter the field. The literature review covers an historical prespective of the occupational segregation of the field; a description of what dance/movement therapy entails; studies of various gender differences; sex role identity and sex role strain theory; a review of the experiences of men in nursing; and a survey of the attitudes of female dance/movement therapists toward male dance/movement therapists.

It was hypothesized that the main deterrents to males entering the field of dance/movement therapy lie outside of any resistance they may encounter from females in the field. The primary deterrents are hypothesized to be sociocultural and economic and are believed to result in strain on males in the field. Questionnaires were sent out to 42 male dance/movement therapists and graduate students. Twenty were completed and returned in time to be used in the present study. Results support the notion that male and female dance/movement therapists have a generally positive relationship. Primary sources of strain are related to occupational status, income, lack of male colleagues and the profession being perceived as violating the male sex role. Primary deterrents to males entering the field appear to be the lack of males with any experience in dance or movement as creative expression. This too appears to be due to sex role socialization and the low status of art in our culture. Recommendations are given about what the profession of dance/movement therapy can do to increase the numbers of men in the field in the long and short term.

Bradshaw, Gail. *Befriending the Body and Rejoining the World: Group Dance/Movement Therapy with Adult Female Incest Survivors within a Partial Hospitalization Program.* Columbia College, 1995.

The purpose of this study was to demonstrate the effectiveness of group dance/movement therapy within a multidisciplinary treatment approach for adult female incest survivors in a partial hospitalization program. Four subjects were followed for their entire length of participation in the partial hospitalization program. After each dance/movement therapy group an observation form was filled out. An assessment was completed and each survivor's progress was evaluated using Marian Chace's principles of therapeutic movement relationship, body action, symbolism and rhythmic group activity. The following three factors were found to influence effectiveness: 1) ability to focus on the body and engage in the movement process 2) stage of healing from the incest experience and 3) the length of involvement in dance/movement therapy. The findings confirm that dance/movement therapy was an effective mode of treatment because the damaged physical and emotional parts of the self are both integrated into the entire healing process. Moreover, since most survivors tend to dissociate from or ignore their physical selves and exhibit poor interpersonal skills, group dance/movement therapy provides a safe and structured way for these survivors to begin befriending their body and rejoining the world.

Brady, Susan. *"The Embodied Organization": A Somatic Approach to Corporate Development.* Naropa Institute, 1996.

A research study was conducted on the effects that movement therapy may have on the psychological, mental and social functioning of individuals working within the corporate arena. Through the development of a somatic-based model for organizational change, movement therapy is tested as a legitimate approach to organizational development, both in principle and practical application. Specifically, this thesis purports that movement therapy will lead to an increased sense of personal empowerment within the corporate organization, as measured by the attributes of autonomy and creativity, two central characteristics of empowerment. Integrating theories of organizational development, it is proposed that the benefits of this somatic-based, individual approach will ultimately be evident on an organizational level.

Bram, Dawn L. *Dance/Movement Therapy and Special Education: A Resource for Employment in Public Schools.* Goucher College, 1993.

The purpose of this project is provide a rationale for dance/movement therapy with special education populations in the public school setting and to provide guidelines and resources for those interested in this work. The literature review addresses most aspects of the integration of special education within the public schools and dance/movement therapy as it relates to this population.

Seven experienced dance/movement therapists working within this setting were interviewed regarding background, the establishment of their present jobs, administrative and clinical aspects, case examples/benefits of dance/movement therapy, recommendations for dance/movement therapists desiring employment including obstacles, areas to emphasize, effective ways to approach the school and additional written and video resources.

The author summarizes the data and includes recommendations made by the therapists and a complete list of their suggested references. It concludes that finances and lack of knowledge are the biggest obstacles to being hired and the recommendations are a valuable source of information to overcome these. Flexibility, creativity and determination are most crucial.

Brandt, Karen. *A Comparative Study of the Dance/Movement Therapy Concepts of Marian Chace and her Students.* Goucher College, 1993.

This is a study of the similarities and differences between Marian Chace and her students in their concepts and practice of dance/movement therapy. It describes Chace's students perceptions of her influence on their work. A review of the literature includes these concepts as well as an historical perspective of the mental health field which may have influenced their work. Students of Chace who are a select group of dance/movement therapy pioneers/clinicians were interviewed.

Results show that in most areas, apparent differences between Chace and her students are primarily due to changes in the mental health field context rather than actual differences in theory and practice. In some areas, it is difficult to assess whether differences are apparent or real because of unclear terminology and discrepancies between what Chace actually practiced and what she wrote. The following is examined: 1) conceptualization of dance/movement therapy as rehabilitation vs psychotherapy; 2) adjunctive vs primary clinical role; 3) intuitive vs systematic approach to treatment; 4) use of verbalizations; 5) use of interactive movement relationship; 6) use of transference phenomena; and 7) patient populations and settings.

The study confirms the relevance and value of Chace's original work to current dance/movement therapy practice of Chace's students and contributes new information about the refinement of Chace's concepts through the work of her students, recognizing their advancements and achievements.

Brauninger, Iris. *Consideration of Children's Held Upper Body Posture as a Reaction to Stressful Events.* Laban Centre for Movement and Dance, 1993.

This thesis focuses on a particular type of upper body posture in children who have been through a number of stressful situations in the past, such as war, separation from their home countries, and arrival as refugees in a new country. The literature was reviewed with regard to the nature and function of upper body posture (UBP), the possible causes of held UBP and the relation to physical and emotional stress, and the conditions which may change and resolve a held UBP.

The case studies of three children who had experienced stressful events as mentioned above, are presented in order to support points made in the literature. It is suggested that a held UBP serves as a bodily defence against stress in children; the conclusion is drawn from both the literature review and the case studies.

Brennan, Erika Rannisto. *Jungian Dance/Movement Therapy and Nondirective Play Therapy: A Treatment Approach to Sexual Aggression in Children.* California State University, Hayward, 1993.

A psychotherapeutic approach to the treatment of sexual aggression in children combines Jungian dance/movement therapy and nondirective play therapy. The technique aims to increase the clients' impulse control, develop clear body boundaries, and decrease needs for power and dominance that these children display.

Dance/movement therapy took place within a school/day treatment center for emotionallly disturbed children and was part of a multidisciplinary system of treatment. Specific techniques used and outcomes are presented through a case vignette. The approach was found to be a viable alternative to the cognitive-behavioral therapies addressed in the literature on sexual aggression. Review of the dance/movement therapy literature focuses on abuse and approaches used with emotionally disturbed children.

Brenner, Traci. *Movement Characteristics of Nontraumatized Latency-Aged Girls: Indentifying Indicators of Sexual Abuse and Other Trauma.* Allegheny University of the Health Sciences (formerly Hahnemann University), 1995.

This thesis field tested a specially designed scale to establish norms in movement characteristics which may be specific to sexually abused, latency-aged girls. This is the first step towards conducting a correlational study between sexually abused girls, otherwise traumatized girls and nontraumatized girls, of latency age. The results lend support to Kestenberg's theory in relation to some of the movement characteristics in latency age. In addition, the findings demonstrate the effectiveness of this scale for latency-age subject groups. Research involving normative data is needed in the field of dance/movement therapy. Established norms are the foundation from which pathology and problems are assessed. Identifying movement characteristics specific to sexually abused, latency-aged girls will aid in the assessment processes of children, in the guidance of treatment planning for dance/movement therapists, and eventually in the detection of child sexual abuse and other trauma. The preliminary nature of this study is stressed and suggestions are made for future research.

Briski, Mika Kamryn. *The Use of Dance/Movement Therapy with Depressed Adolescents.* University of California, Los Angeles, 1995. (SP)

Brodersohn, Alicia. *The Pychological, Artistic and Social Changes Which May Have Influenced Marian Chace.* Goucher College, 1993.

This literature review describes the influences of the early twentieth century that seemed to have created an atmosphere conducive to Chace's molding of the principles, goals and process of dance/movement therapy. The literature of psychology, the arts (especially dance) and the social context of the period are reviewed. The innovations of Freudian psychoanalysis, Sullivan's interpersonal theory, Moreno's psychodrama and the emergence of group therapy are discussed. The ideas and underlying philosophy of Chace's teachers of dance, Ruth St. Denis, Ted Shawn and Jacques Dalcroze are examined along with how modern dance appears to have contributed to the fundamentals on which dance/movement therapy is based with its connection to emotional expression, its social meaning and its values for communication. This, combined with the economic and social changes that resulted from World War II, creating changes in the treatment of psychiatric illness and in the redefining of women's roles, became the basis for the psychotherapeutic use of dance.

Brower, Diane. *The Role of Play in Dance Therapy with Adults.* Naropa Institute, 1994.

The focus of this thesis is to examine what play is and what its functions are. With this information as a guide, play is compared to dance therapy in an attempt to determine how play is therapeutic and how it can be used in therapy, particularly dance therapy, with adults.

Brown, Kimeri. *The Individual Dance: Children's Body Image and Self-Identity in Dance/Movement Therapy.* Naropa Institute, 1991.

This thesis explores the relationship between children's body image and sense of self. By working on children's body image development with dance therapy techniques, this thesis hypothesizes that children's sense of self can be enhanced.

The review of literature contains information on the development of self-concept, body image formation and function, the relationship between body image and sense of self, disturbances in body image and how dance therapy works with the body image developmental process.

Three case studies of preschool age children have also been included. Two of these children have developmental disabilities. One child has no extra developmental challenges. The case studies document each child's developmental level in regards to body image and sense of self. The studies describe how dance therapy techniques were used and there is a comparison of draw-a-person tests to describe the progress made by the children.

The conclusion discusses the interrelationship between body image, sense of self, and dance therapy. Suggestions are made for further research.

Brown, Paula J. *The Development of Dance/Movement Therapy Assessment of the Literature as Related to 400 Years of Schizophrenia in the History of Medical Psychology.* Allegheny University of the Health Sciences (formerly Hahnemann University), 1991.

This literature review was undertaken in an attempt to discover if the current theories of the treatment of schizophrenia and the current practice of dance/movement therapy interface. The question asked is: has dance/movement therapy integrated new information about schizophrenia into its practice or has the field continued to operate under assumptions established earlier in its development? Results revealed that overall, based on practitioners chosen, current theory of the etiology of schizophrenia and the clinical practice of movement therapy interface. It also appears that dance/movement therapy's development was due to its timeliness. A review of current literature underscored the importance of the field of movement therapy keeping abreast of current scientific research in order to ensure the survival of the field. It was also apparent that the current economic situation requires increased sophistication from its clinicians and continued incorporation of new findings.

Browne, W. Ruthe. *Wholeness and Holiness Restored Through Dance: Applictions of Sacred Dance Movement Therapy.* Columbia College, 1990.

The beginning of the search for wholeness and holiness through dance therapy led to sacred dance. The desire to re-experience wholeness using sacred dance movements led me to search for a therapeutic counterpart in treating patients. Dance therapy uses movement to bring about physical and psychic integration. The psychic includes mind, soul, and the spirit; yet the spiritual aspect has not been overtly integrated into dance therapy.

This thesis demonstrates how dance/movement therapy can help the patient become aware of and learn to integrate transpersonal dimensions of one's psyche for the purpose of deepening and completing one's quest for wholeness in an unconscious search for completion and meaning to one's life. This transcendent dimension includes unconscious material, archetypes, and synchronized events experienced in the environment.

Bryson, Rosalyn Cundy. *Inviting Conscious Ritual into the Field of Dance Therapy: An Exploration of the Healing Qualities of Ritual and Authentic Movement.* Naropa Institute, 1994.

This thesis explores authentic movement as a form of ritual that has healing potential in the field of dance therapy. It is suggested that authentic movement provides the opportunity for participants to embody their individuality in a supportive community that also fosters learning about self and other. The idea of learning about self and other by emphasizing the value in seeing another human being, being seen by another and ultimately seeing the self will be developed through the study of authentic movement and through research on ritual in other cultures.

The review of literature contains information on dance therapy, ritual, and movement ritual. Emphasis will be placed on the role that ritual/movement ritual has in creating community and in learning about self and other. The discussion explores authentic movement as a ritual and as a state of being. It is in this section that the interface between authentic movement and dance therapy is addressed. The thesis contains five interviews with people who have experienced authentic movement. Suggestions for further research are also included.

Bunce, Jillian Margery. *Dance Movement Therapy with Groups of Parkinson's Disease Patients and their Carers.* Laban Centre London, 1996.

This thesis is an attempt to describe dance movement therapy with Parkinson's disease patients and their carers. The author looks at posture and its relevance to the therapeutic process and its relationship to the pathology of the disease. These elements provide metaphors for the psychological dynamics used in the creative process in the therapy.

A description of the pathology of the disease highlights the relevance of the importance of body and posture to the movement process. It indicates the importance of movement analysis and how it is relevant to dance movement therapy with Parkinson's patients. It assesses the benefits of dance movement therapy from questionnaires and includes case vignettes.

This thesis is based on work with Parkinson's Disease patients at a small hospital in the midlands. The work began in September 1992 and continues at present. The work and the context in which it took place is described and it is suggested that further research could quantify the benefits of dance movement therapy with Parkinson's disease patients.

Burden, Kimberley A. *Further Research into The Interface of the Kestenberg Movement Profile and Body-Mind Centering(TM): An Examination of Common Ground Between The Tension Flow Rhythms and The Qualities of The Physiological Fluids.* Antioch/New England Graduate School, 1995.

An examination of the parallels between the Kestenberg Movement Profile (KMP) Tension Flow Rhythms and the fluid systems of Body-Mind Centering(tm) (BMC) is presented. Fifty-eight BMC practitioners recorded their observations of fluid qualities present in the performance of the ten KMP Tension Flow Rhythms (TFRs). The results are presented and discussed in light of implications and existing literature relevant to the KMP, BMC, and body-mind psychology. Consistent responses to the observational study are discussed and suggestions are made for application to clinical work. Recommendations are made for further study in the areas of additional observation and notation to encourage cross-fertilization of the two systems, as well as for further research concerning the physiological implications of the interface of the TFRs and fluid systems in service of the advancement of body-mind studies.

Burns, Carolyn. *Object Relations Dance/Movement Therapy and Attention in Children with Attention Deficit.* Antioch/New England Graduate School, 1995.

This thesis explores the use of regressive object relations dance/movement therapy as an intervention tool with children diagnosed with attention deficit disorder and attention deficit with hyperactivity. This paper uses developmental, essential psychodynamic literature as its base. The study is a single case study of a four year old boy diagnosed with attention deficit/hyperactivity. The Kestenberg Movement Profile provides the measurement tool for the study. Possible implications for dance/movement therapists are discussed in the final chapter.

Burns, Frances. *A Dance/Movement Therapy Model for Working with Children.* California State University, Hayward, 1993.

This study creates a treatment model for the use of dance/movement therapy with children who exhibit emotional/behavioral disturbance. This treatment model emphasizes the role of environment in supporting the healing process. An awareness of social and emotional contexts in which the child is embedded increases the effectiveness of the therapist's interventions.

Burt, John W. Body. *Face, and Voice: Nonverbal Expression of Emotion in Infancy.* Creative Arts in Therapy Program and Ph.D. Clinical Psychology Program, Allegheny University of the Health Sciences (formerly Hahnemann University), 1995.

Ever since the work of Charles Darwin, there has been scientific inquiry into the nonverbal expression of emotion. Especially in the past 25 years, evidence for specific constellations of emotional signals has been accumulating. Whereas patterns of facial expression of many basic emotions have been well established, there is insufficient objective research into the vocal and body movement signals of the fundamental affect states. The study hypothesized that there are specific combinations of vocal and body movement signals that co-exist with facial expression constellations. Eighty segments of 13-month old infants displaying facial expressions of joy, interest, sadness, or anger were coded for the simultaneously occurring vocal and body movement signals of emotion. Vocalization parameters including phase length, volume, pitch range, and harmonic tone were found to distinguish the emotions. Body movement indicators of emotion included the changing of the body shape in space, and the quality of shifts in muscular tension. Conclusions support the differential emotions theory (Izard, 1972).

Callaghan, Karen. *Movement Psychotherapy with Torture Survivors.* Laban Centre for Movement and Dance, 1991.

Case, Valinda. *Relevance of Body Memories Relived in a Dance/Movement Therapy Context with Traumatized Patients.* University of California, Los Angeles, 1994. (SP)

Cerami, Francesca. *Formerly Battered Women: Healing of the Self Through Dance/Movement Therapy.* New York University, 1992.

This study was designed as a quasi-experiment utilizing dance/movement therapy to facilitate the healing process of formerly battered women. It was designed to explore whether dance/movement therapy is a viable treatment tool to facilitate change in formerly battered women's relationship to her body, and consequently her self. Included was exploration of whether dance/movement therapy may foster a) an awareness of the body and self, b) integration of the body and self and c) acceptance of the body and self. The findings confirmed that this population may benefit from dance/movement therapy to aid in developing a relationship between the body and the self to foster wholeness and healing from domestic violence crisis.

Champlin, Kate. *Resistance: How To Work with it in Contemplative Somatic Dance/Movement Therapy.* Naropa Institute, 1995.

This thesis hypothesizes that resistance in the therapeutic process can be effectively worked through by means of Contemplative Somatic Dance/Movement Therapy. The described therapy is a combination of contemplative, somatic, and dance/movement therapies. In proving the hypothesis, each of the three schools of psychotherapy is described separately and an integration is constructed. Effectiveness of the integrative method in working with resistance is supported with examples from nine interviews with therapists who work in the fields of contemplative, somatic, and dance/movement therapies.

The literature review includes primary theories and methods used by each psychotherapeutic school, the concept of self and theories and methods for working with resistance utilized by each. Examples are given. The conclusion restates how the integration of contemplative, somatic, and dance/movement therapies offers an effective means for working with resistance in the therapeutic process. Limitations to the empirical study are stated and suggestions for further study.

Chapek, Kathleen. *Improvisation as a Tool within the Dance Process.* California State University, Hayward, 1991.

This project examined the effects of improvisation in dance and to document the process and its psycho-social impact on adolescents (includes 30 minute video). A three month program provided formal dance structures along with imagery and movement exercises to encourage in-depth self-exploration and self-expression. Verbalization and discussion was structured as part of experience so that the process allowed exploration of improvisational movement and emotions connected to it.

Chenier, Karen Bruce. *Use of Imagery with Traumatized Adult Holocaust Survivors in Dance/Movement Therapy Groups.* University of Califormia, Los Angeles, 1996. (SP)

Chessman, Paula. *The Integration of Dance Therapy into the Practice of Psychiatric Rehabilitation.* Hunter College 1993.

The author suggests what dance therapists must do in order to integrate the concepts and practice of psychiatric rehabilitation into dance therapy methodology. There is a synthesis of existing literature in the fields of dance/movement therapy and psychiatric rehabilitation with chronic schizophrenic patients, and the author's experiences as a dance/movement therapist in a Psychiatric Rehabilitation setting at South Beach Psychiatric Center (SBPC). An attempt is made to describe what it is about the pyschiatric rehabilitation system as practiced at SBPC that is presently incongruent to the practice of dance/movement therapy; the areas in which these two fields seem to share commonalities in the areas of treatment processes, principles and philosophy; and what would have to change in order to successfully integrate dance/movement therapy into the system at South Beach.

Chutroo, Barbara. *Anxiety: A Theoretical Overview and Personal Account.* Hunter College, 1991.

This paper presents a theoretical overview and personal account of anxiety. Anxiety's causes are discussed, particularly its origins in childhood experiences. A case study is presented of my own experiences with anxiety in relation to authority during my progress through and beyond the Hunter College Dance/Movement Therapy program.

Chyorny, Raisa. *Using Dance/Movement and Other Creative Therapies in a Teacher Support Program.* Naropa Institute, 1995.

This thesis proposes a teacher support program which uses techniques of dance/movement and other creative arts therapies. Four questions are investigated. 1) Is a teacher support program necessary for the well-being of educational institutions? 2) Will a teacher support program be endorsed by the members of an educational institution? 3) Are the methods of creative arts therapies appropriate for a teacher support program? 4) Does individual growth propel the social system toward positive change?

The results are obtained using preliminary questionnaires, literature reviews, pilot studies, observation, and direct communication with teachers. Extensive literature reviews of education and dance/movement therapy are presented followed by detailed descriptions of three pilot studies conducted in St. Petersburg, Russia. The pilot studies are conducted in the context of a creative arts therapies conference, an orphanage, and a public school.

The results suggest affirmation of questions 1, 2, and 3. There is not enough information to answer question 4.

Clarke, Margaret S. *Psychodynamic Dance/Movement Therapy with Obsessive-Compulsive Disorders.* Antioch/New England Graduate School, 1991.

This thesis presents the view that dance/movement therapy is an excellent modality for treating obsessive-compulsive disorders. To this end, the author examines the intra-psychic structure of the obsessive-compulsive personality in order to clarify how the body as a container for the self is instrumental in the manifestation of this disease. Through incorporating dance/movement therapy and other therapies, the author explores the ways in which the body has been incorporated into treatment. Dance/movement therapy (DMT) is described as applied to the treatment of several individuals suffering from various obsessive-compulsive disorders. The use of DMT is believed to have had a positive impact on the healing process of each individual treated.

Clauer, Melanie. *The Application of Dance/Movement Therapy with TJ: A Suicidal Eight Year Old Boy.* University of California, Los Angeles, 1993.

This thesis provides an illustrative case study of work with a suicidal child within the dance/movement therapy treatment framework. Research finds there to be no current information specific to the application of the dance-therapy process. Thus, a purpose of this study is to increase the body of literature on the childhood suicidal phenomenon.

A historical review of the literature concerning depression, it's origin and treatment, and its role as an antecedent to suicidal behavior is provided. Dr. Cynthia Pfeffer, a leading researcher in this area, developed a three phase approach to dealing with suicidal children. The interventions she applies are based on psychoanalytic theory, and emphasize issues surrounding attachment, loss, and separation. A discussion of the applicability of Pfeffer's approach, finds that most of the goals and interventions proposed easily transfer to the dance/movement treatment setting. Overall it was felt by this therapist that Pfeffer's model provides a firm foundation for the dance-therapy process.

Coburn, Letitia. *Experiencing and Transforming: Dance Therapy Imagery of an HIV+ Client.* Hunter College, 1995.

This paper analyzes the use of dance/movement therapy (DMT) to explore the movement and imagery of a client with three diagnoses: schizophrenia, crack addiction and an HIV+ status. Grounded in the work of Kubler-Ross and Jung, the research utilizes both quantitative and qualitative approaches. The client's movement and imagery are examined to assess her degree of "experiencing." Degree of "experiencing" (Gendlin) is determined via a quantitative analysis of the level of the imagery (Lusebrink) and the accompanying movement's point of initiation in the body.

The client's degree of "experiencing" increases as the DMT work progresses and after discussion (between therapist and client) of the client's HIV+ status. The imagery is analyzed qualitatively from a Jungian perspective and reveals themes related to transformation, and death and dying. Suggestions are made to facilitate further research into DMT with people with AIDS and to improve clinical practice with this same population.

Cohen, Amy E. *A Personal "Dual Degree" Synthesis: A Comparison of the Theory and Practice of Dance/Movement Therapy and Nonverbal Methods of Social Group Work.* Hunter College, 1994.

This paper compares the theory and practice of dance/movement therapy and activity groups in social work in order to synthesize the knowledge gained in a dual degree program combining these two disciplines. Grounded in systems thinking, a cohesive approach to groups is developed which encompasses both verbal and nonverbal aspects of communication. A review of the literature contrasts the theoretical similarities and differences of purpose, goals, methods, healing processes, phases of group development, and the role of the leader. A dance/movement therapy group and an arts and crafts group at a day treatment center for adults diagnosed mentally ill are then analyzed to explore how the related concepts are enacted in practice. Similarities are noted in each discipline's assumption that a sense of self and an ability to relate to others develops within the stream of human action and group relationships.

The resulting analysis found differences in three areas of practice: 1) pregroup planning, 2) use of nonverbal communication, and 3) role taken in relation to the group. Whereas highly organized and prescriptive structuring led to success in the social work activities group, the process of dance therapy demanded "informed spontaneity" as a form of pregroup planning. In addition, although both methods utilized symbolic forms of communication in conjunction with discussion, training in dance/movement therapy enabled the leader to understand the meaning inherent in body movement, and to provide insight by crystallizing the group's experience physically. This nonverbal mode of interaction placed a greater emphasis on the mutual and reciprocal aspects of the leader-group relationship.

Cohen Joanne. *Dance/Movment Therapy in Israel.* University of California, Los Angeles, 1993. (SP)

Comer, Matthew E. *Dance Therapy and Gay Men with AIDS.* Hunter College, 1992.

This thesis examines the use of dance therapy interventions with a population of "normal neurotic" gay men that are HIV positive or are in the symptomatic stages of AIDS. The history of male homosexuality, its predominance in society and society's response to homosexuality is reviewed. The progression of the disease from HIV seropositivity to AIDS is focused on as well as the effect of AIDS on body and mental functioning. Also examined is the public response to HIV/AIDS and an overview of group work that has been done with this population.

Comyn, Ana Ruiz-Benetez de Lugo. *The Relationship Between Impulse Control and Sign Language Mastery in Deaf Children: a Pilot Study.* Laban Centre for Movement and Dance, 1993.

Connell, Jean. *Movement Therapy for the Angry Adolescent.* Hunter College, 1991.

The primary goal of this thesis is to provide a model for treating the angry adolescent in dance/movement therapy. In constructing this model, the author incorporates the ideas of anger-control management from a cognitive-behavioral perspective. There is a review recognizing adolescent self-concept as theorized by E.H. Erikson. A case study is presented which includes many movement suggestions for dealing with the adolescent and his/her impulsive aggressive reaction to anger. This case-study will demonstrate that in order for an adolescent to control aggressive-impulsive behavior they must possess some recognition of self.

Connolly, Kimberly. *An Assessment of Body Attitude in Four Individuals with Multiple Personality Disorder.* Allegheny University of the Health Sciences (formerly Hahnemann University), 1994.

This study of body attitude of four individuals with Multiple Personality Disorder hypothesized that each personality will have different movement characteristics, while transitions between personalities will have greater variation. Twelve raters rated eight separate personalities to determine the absence or presence of variables of body attitude. The dependent measures were alignment in space, body shaping, postural shaping in planes, use of posture and gesture and areas of tension. Inter-rated reliability ranged from zero to 90% agreement. The data provided promising support of the hypothesis and indicates the need for future research in this area.

Connors, Joan. *An Investigation into The Parallels in The Healing Process Between Dance/Movement Therapy and Sacred Circle Dance.* Antioch/New England Graduate School, 1994.

Sacred circle dance is a ritualized dance form based on folk and ethnic dances which embody characteristics of ancient healing dances. These dances provided communities through the ages with a technique for healing the psyche. Dance movement therapy is a psychotherapeutic healing modality in which body movement can promote health and growth. This thesis examines the parallels in the healing processes in both sacred circle dance and dance/movement therapy utilizing the eight healing processes that Claire Schmais has identified in group dance therapy as a basis for comparison. The similar organizing features: synchrony, rhythm and the circular formation are explored. The comparable functions including the creation of community, diminishment of isolation, the transformative process and symbolic significance are discussed. An investigation into the history of both forms provides a common root. The use of sacred circle dances in dance/ movement therapy groups is examined and both the positive and negative aspects of including a structured ritual form in an improvisational style of dance movement/ therapy groups are presented.

Conwell, Donna. *Dance/Movement Therapy as an Approach to the Integration of Body Image with Individuals Sustaining Traumatic Brain Injury: A Synthesis of Literature.* Allegheny University of the Health Sciences (formerly Hahnemann University), 1991.

With advances in acute and post-acute care, the number of survivors of traumatic brain injury (TBI) are on the rise. This thesis reviews and synthesizes the literature of TBI, body image and its role in the process of rehabilitation. It supports dance/movement therapy as a tool for integration of self through the body with individuals surviving TBI. The author concludes that existing literature is supportive of the dance/movement therapy as a tool for integration of both the past and presently held sense of self through the body with the TBI patient. Research indicates that survivors must adapt to cognitive, physical, and emotional changes in the self due to losses experienced as a result of the injury. Recovery appears to be developmental in nature and seems best facilitated by a multi-model approach. Clients frequently describe the integration of previous and presently held body image through body referenced statements, either verbal or nonverbal (loss of verbal articulation to expressfeelings is common with these individuals). The body is a universal reference point for the sensory experience and understanding of "self". The brain helps to organize and make meaning of body level experiences on both conscious and unconscious levels. It appears that a psychological experience occurs in harmony with physical and cognitive processes. It is with this event the emotions become connected to the formation of one's sense of self in the world.

Cooper, Audrey C. *An Exploratory Look at the Dance/Movement Therapist's Role and Practice with a Group of Deaf Adolescents.* Hunter College, 1995.

This paper describes the differential role and practice requirements of the dance/movement therapist working with adolescents who are deaf. A review of the literature reveals the historical reporting of pervasive social-emotional and behavioral problems for deaf youth. These behaviors are reframed by both a human developmental perspective which recognizes common biopsychosocial stressors of the adolescent period, as well as by a sociocultural perspective which recognizes the often misunderstood cultural and linguistic behaviors of the deaf community.

The dance/movement therapist's role and practice with one group of deaf adolescents is described to illuminate group needs and practice responses. Similarities and differences are noted between working with hearing and deaf populations, respectively. Whereas actual dance/movement therapy activities and group development were found to unfold in an average expectable way, major differences were noted in the areas of communication mode, transmitting messages/cuing, use of music, lights, and props, and verbal (signed) processing. Dance therapy practice with hearing persons typically relies upon the use of music and the ability to call out directions while movement exploration is carried out. With deaf individuals, colorful props were found to provide the emotional shading and stimulation that music provides to the hearing. In addition, to transmit messages, American Sign Language, a visual-manual language, requires conversants to make eye contact presenting challenges to the therapist who, in promoting immersion in an activity or movement experience, must find alternate ways to impart information without inhibiting the mover/participant.

Cornwall, Rebecca Patricia. *Facilitating Positive Social Experiences with Internalizing and Externalizing Special Needs Children through Group Dance/Movement Therapy: A Pilot Study.* University of California, Los Angeles, 1992.

Many special needs children experience difficulties in social situations. Although the etiology of these difficulties varies from child to child, persistent socialization problems in childhood often lead to a number of affective and adjustment problems in adolescence and adulthood. The affective and adjustment disorders experienced in later life interfere not only with an individual's social experiences, but also interfere with employment, schooling, and one's overall sense of selfworth.

This pilot study explores the facilitation of positive social experiences for special needs children with internalizing and externalizing behavior styles. Thirty-one elementary school students from a private school for children with academic, behavioral and emotional difficulties participated in the study. The students experienced eight adapted dance/movement therapy sessions which were each designed to emphasize one of three social structures; working individually, in pairs, or as a group. Each session was evaluated by the students as well as by the therapist/researcher.

The findings indicate that while internalizers preferred the individual social structure and the externalizers preferred the group social structure, both behavior style categories were found significantly more appealing by their peers while involved in the individual social structured sessions. These findings are discussed in terms of their usefulness in designing dance/movement therapy interventions which more appropriately and successfully facilitate positive social experiences with this population of children.

Correa, Marcela. *The Creation and Performance/Exhibition of an Artistic Piece as a Therapeutic Process (Working Approach and Case Studies in Dance Therapy).* Lesley College Graduate School, 1992.

This thesis investigates the course of creating an artistic piece and the act of performing or exhibiting the final creation as a therapeutic process. This approach was investigated within the field of dance/movement therapy. The work was conducted with two populations: normal adult females, including the author; and preadolescent and adolescent multiple-handicapped, blind/low vision adolescents and young adults. With the normal adult population, the work was based on Authentic Movement. With special needs individuals, the original Authentic Movement approach was fit to each case or group. Other expressive methods were explored as an adjunct to dance/movement therapy such as story writing and art. Six case studies are included detailing examples of the different populations worked with.

Cowen, Helena. *Object Relations and Jungian Theories of Symbol Formation and their Relevance to Dance Movement Therapy with Children.* Laban Centre for Movement and Dance, 1993.

Crowley, Rebecca. *Dance/Movement Therapy With a Frail Elderly Population.* Lesley College Graduate School, 1992.

This thesis describes dance/movement groups with a frail elderly population at the writer's internship site. The concepts of Marion Chace are explained, and the benefits of dance/movement therapy for elderly people are discussed. There are journal entries which describe the writer's personal and professional process as well as reflections, dreams, and poetry about aging.

Cruz, Robyn Flaum. *An Empirical Investigation of the Movement Psychodiagnostic Inventory.* University of Arizona, 1995. (Doctoral)

Abnormal motor behavior associated with psychopathology was investigated in this study using a nontraditional inventory, the Movement Psychodiagnostic Inventory, with a sample of psychiatric patients that included personality disorders and individuals with schizophrenia and schizophrenia spectrum disorders. The study was designed to address several methodolgical and measurement problems noted in the literature, and to this end ratings were made from videotaped observations allowing detection of subtle movements described in terms of their dynamic, spatial, rhythmic and muscular involvement rather than labeled with traditional terminology.

Parameters of nonverbal communicative behavior were also rated. Although diagnostic groups not associated with disturbed motor behavior were included, univariate analysis failed to reveal differences between diagnostic groups with a long history of association with abnormal motor behavior and those without such a history. Multidimensional scaling and cluster analysis were thus employed to uncover the structure of the data in exploratory analyses that used two distance measures and several methods each of multidimensional scaling and cluster analysis. Results were interpreted to indicate that different patterns of movement behavior were observed for each group of patients that were not measure-or- method dependent. The results of the study are discussed within the context of the potential for the inventory and the advancement of the study of motor behavior and psychopathology, an area that has the potential to effect progress in diagnosis, etiology, pathogenesis, and treatment of mental disorders.

Curtin, Patti. *The Moon and Movement Therapy.* Antioch/New England Graduate School, 1994.

This thesis is a theoretical synthesis of astrological, spiritual and feminist perspective of the impact of the Moon and its myths on the psyche. I have combined this synthesis with the Kestenberg Movement Profile for the purpose of application to dance/movement therapy theory and practice.

Curtis Sue. *The Use of Play in a Non-directive Approach to Dance Movement Therapy.* Laban Centre for Movement and Dance, 1993.

Daigle, Rollande. *Application of the Kestenberg Movement Profile to the Clinical Assessment of The Mother-Autistic Child Dyad.* Antioch/New England Graduate School, 1993.

This is a case study of a mother-child dyad in which the Kestenberg Movement Profile is used as a methodological tool to assess the progress and efficacy of a dance/movement therapy treatment for early childhood autism. During five months, eleven dance/movement therapy sessions involving the mother and her child were videotaped. Complete Kestenberg Movement Profiles of the child and mother during the pre-(first video) and post-tests (last video) were drawn and analyzed. The pre-test and post-test performances were then compared and discussed in terms of attunement and clashing in the mother-child interaction. The profiles of the dyad were analyzed step-by-step and discussed in relation to this question: Which KMP factors will be retained as relevant in evaluating the effect of the treatment on a mother-autistic child dyad? The results reveal that the KMP has the potential to delimit very precisely the areas of conflict and harmony at both the personal and relational levels.

Danner, Jennifer. *Dance/Movement Therapy in a Multicultural High School Context.* University of California, Los Angeles, 1994.(SP)

Davies, Mary I. *Setting Up a Programme of Movement Therapy in a Mainstream London Primary School.* Laban Centre for Movement and Dance, 1992.

Davis, Annica. *Case Study of an Autistic Child.* Antioch/New England Graduate School. 1991.

This thesis investigates the impact of dance/movement therapy on the symptomatic functioning of a pre-school age autistic child. The techniques and interventions described here grew out of a context of psychoanalytically-oriented dance/movement therapy, based on object relations and developmental theories. The unfolding therapeutic process is viewed along those theoretical lines. Several constructs and concepts shared by both psychoanalysis and dance/movement therapy are discussed along with the viability of their applications. The literature reviewed is of those theorists whose views have strongly influenced the writer.

Davis, Consuelo V. *Nommotion: An African-Centered Model of Dance Movement Therapy.* University of California, Los Angeles, 1993.

Dance movement therapy is presented from an African-centered perspective which provides a comprehensive, culturally sensitive treatment model for Africans in the United States. Research indicates that significant differences exist in the cultural worldview perceptions of African and

European Americans, and that African Americans may experience unique circumstances which historically have not been acknowledged, understood, or addressed, in the field of psychotherapy. As a result, African American psychologists have endeavored to implement treatment methodologies which create strategies to address their clients' psychological needs and redefine the social structure to be fundamentally supportive of Africans in the United States.

The author has developed the Nommotion, African-centered model of dance movement therapy (N'ACDMT) which is based on the theoretical methods and values of dance movement therapy, African psychology, and the African centered philosophical worldview perspectives. This paradigm integrates elements of expressive movement, Nommo (the generative power of word-force), ethos, spirituality, creativity, rhythm, and culturally sensitive therapeutic interventions, so that clients may be informed on multiple channels of universal self/Self consciousness in a culturally familiar environment. The N'ACDMT model suggests interventions which enhance clients' propensity towards self/Self help and self/Self actualization, and has been applied to six African American women in Los Angeles, California. Based on the reports of the participants and the writer (as a participant observer) the impact of the N'ACDMT model has been described and documented, and provides the foundation for future research.

DeArment, Mary. *Movement Characteristics of an Individual with Multiple Personality Disorder.* Allegheny University of the Health Sciences (formerly Hahnemann University), 1993.

This single subject research project presents an analysis of the movement characteristics of a subject diagnosed with Multiple Personality Disorder. Four pairs of raters, blind to the study, watched the videotape without sound and scored occurrence, incidence, or duration of designated movement parameters (head position, gaze, postural system, gesticulation, foot action, hand fidgets, and chair swivel). Inter-rater reliability varied from nil to 98%. The researcher and senior nonverbal behavior research advisor analyzed the data for patterns. "Movement states" were identified that were found to correspond to the emergence of alters (personalities) as verbally identified by the subject. Additionally, two movement patterns persisted throughout each altered state. Correlations between verbal content and movement states are discussed.

De Beer, Edna. *Using Dance Therapy with Psychoactive Substance Users To Change Patterns of Mechanisms For Coping.* Hunter College, 1992.

The purpose of this thesis is to explore the relationship between coping mechanisms and dependent psychoactive substance use. The ability to engage adaptive coping mechanisms is related to positive feelings of self-esteem and self-efficacy. The development of these processes is investigated. Dance therapy is introduced as an adjunctive therapy to assist in the rehabilitation process. Through movement the dependent psychoactive substance user can develop a clearer and more positive sense of self. This process should enhance feelings of self-esteem and self-efficacy which will enable the development of adaptive coping mechanisms.

DeJean, Denise. *Bembe: A Healing Experience.* Hunter College, 1994.

This thesis discusses the relationship between bembe and dance therapy, and discusses the importance of myth and ritual in the life of an individual. A theory is developed using a cultural ritual to expand theories of dance therapy in order to meet the needs of an existing community within the mental health care system made up of third world peoples and cultures.

It has been understood that for ancient peoples, myth and ritual are intrinsic to their experience of themselves and their universe. Ritual was the expression of myth in a physical form. Community rituals were directed towards healing, sustenance, and cohesion. These experiences were choreographed by the chief healing agent, the shaman.

In urban centers of the modern world healing continues to occur, using rituals that have come down from ancient times to current days. Bembe, is one such ritual. It connects the individual to the universe by allowing the deities to align first with the individual, and then with the community through the process of possession and cleansing. Dance therapy is another form of healing, that connects the body/mind of an individual to themselves and then to the community of humanity. Both of these are working towards the same goal of healing of the individual with the community.

DeJesus, Michelle. *Discriminating Movement Behaviors of Adult Psychotic Patients due to Medication Effects vs. Psychopathology.* University of California, Los Angeles, 1993. (SP)

DeLeon, Frances. *Dance/Movement Therapy: A Treatment Modality for the Therapeutic Issues Arising from a Near-Death Experience.* University of California, Los Angeles, 1994. (SP)

Diaz-Salazar, Pepi. *Dancing My Life.* Hunter College, 1992.

This study centers upon the dance experience I shared with a fellow student over the course of a year and a half. During this time I tried to answer for myself the questions as to what the dance in dance/movement therapy was: what is the reality of a dance experience on a personal level, why I feel the need to dance? In answering these questions for myself, I have drawn upon the wisdom of dancers, dance critics, dance/movement therapists, psychologists, philosophers, poets and writers, intertwining their writings with the dances they illuminated for me.

Dillian, Carolyn Elizabeth. *The Professional Status of Dance/Movement Therapy.* Goucher College, 1991.

Through a questionnaire format, dance/movement therapists and professionals working with dance/movement therapists were questioned about perceptions of the professional status of dance/movement therapy. Demographic information, selected questions and responses on the Interprofessional Perceptions Scale (IPS) were analyzed. The IPS, developed by Golin and Ducanis (1981), determines relationships from three perspectives: 1) the respondent's viewpoint, 2) the respondent's view of how an other professional would answer, and 3) the respondent's view of how the other professional would say he/she (i.e., the respondent) answered. Questions for dance/movement therapy professionals were designed to elicit qualitative, personal impressions of the status of dance/movement therapists. Questions for non-dance/movement therapy professionals were designed to elicit impressions of the status of dance/movement therapists, as well as to assess the interprofessional knowledge concerning dance/movement therapists.

Literature reviewed included sociological conceptualizations of professions and socialization into a professional role, and historical, clinical and professional aspects of dance/movement therapy.

Three conclusions, based upon the literature, the IPS, and the questionnaire, can be made from this research. It is indicated that people in the dance/ movement therapy profession are competent, caring and ethical; however, comparative information (between groups) indicated that differences in perceptions do occur in some interdisciplinary areas: encroachment, defensiveness, autonomy and the utilization of the capabilities of other professionals. Information gleaned from the questionnaires was rather positive and includes four main conclusions: 1) dance/movement therapy is seen as a necessary modality, 2) the budgetary constraints of facilities was often mentioned as possibly affecting dance/

movement therapy's presence in a facility, 3) dance/movement therapists self-report educating other professionals to attain a professional image, and 4) non-dance/movement therapists report the primary method of attaining interprofessional knowledge concerning dance/movement therapy is through personal contact with a dance/movement therapist.

Dillman, Deborah S. *Somatic-Expressive Group Process as a Tool Toward Healing the Wounding of Childhood in Adolescents.* Naropa Institute, 1995.

An experiential group process which embraces somatic, reflective and expressive therapeutic modalities has the potential to improve self-awareness, self-acceptance, self-expression, social awareness and healthful social behavior in adolescents. These characteristics are essential parameters of the psychological healing process.

The progress of twenty-eight adolescents, ages 13 to 16, was followed over the course of eight therapeutic sessions, scheduled twice a week for four weeks. Each of these students had been given a DSM-3 psychiatric diagnosis and had been legally assigned to a residential adolescent treatment facility prior to this study. Their length of residence in this facility ranged from 6 months to several years.

Goals of the study included an increase in self-awareness, self-acceptance and self-expression, enhancing skills in relating to self and others, and an improvement in their ability to exhibit both healthful autonomy and cooperation. It is significant that shifts did occur during the one-month trial period of somatic-expressive therapeutic groups. In certain clients and indicators, the changes were more evident than in others. The need for this work to continue over a longer period of time is apparent.

DiNoto, Linda Marie. *Dance Therapy/Group Therapy: Theory and Practice.* Naropa Institute, 1990.

This paper grew out of an increasing need to define and clarify what the author was trying to do as a dance therapist. Attracted to the field of dance therapy because she saw dance as capturing the beauty and vividness that is inherent in human form and motion, dance therapy seemed like an innovative way of combining an interest in the hidden or invisible aspects of human nature with an interest in the expressive arts. As time went on, she came to realize that dance therapy, as a practice, is not so much a form that one learns, as a form that one develops by synthesizing one's own connection to movement and to psychotherapy.

DiPalma, Eleanor Maria. *Liljan Winifred Espenak, Pioneer: Her Life and Work in the Profession of Dance Therapy.* New York University, 1993. (Doctoral)

This is an examination of the life and work of Liljan Espenak (1905-1988) and her primary place in the context of dance/movement therapy as an emerging profession. Information regarding Espenak's life and work was gleaned from personal interviews with Espenak's colleagues and former students, mail surveys, books, articles, and other sources. Twenty two students and five colleagues presented in-depth descriptions of Espenak's character, her style of relating to her peers, students and patients, her clinical approach, and her dance therapy training approach. Nine present and past officers of the American Dance Therapy Association responded to an ADTA survey. Several elements of Espenak's conceptual framework are highlighted including the discovery by this author in Espenak's notes and manuscript of a later conceptualization of Espenak's involving an in-depth look at the relationship of psyche and soma as revealed in the human walk.

In addition to substantiating Espenak's professional contributions and influence in dance/

movement therapy, this study shows that her pioneering efforts were not fully realized by a profession that, still in flux, is struggling to further its place in the United States.

Dolin, Julie E. *Rhythmic Movement as a Formative Process: Its Influence on Sense of Time and Sense of Self.* Naropa Institute, 1991.

This thesis explores the hypothesis that a personal sense of time cultivated through awareness of our internal, rhythmic processes and in response to nature is an integral part of sense of self and prepares us for satisfying relationships. Literature review includes biological rhythms, the space-time model of physics, pre- and peri-natal imprints and the child's developing sense of time, interaction rhythms, the Buddhist concept of being in the moment, rhythm in healing rituals, and the use of rhythm in dance/movement therapy. The author advocates a paradigm shift from an externally imposed, primarily linear sense of time to a sense of time based upon a fluctuating response to an internal reference point. Three research groups—two on an inpatient psychiatric unit, one with compulsive over-eaters—serve as experiments in D/MT techniques for beginning this shift.

Dripchak, Valerie. *Improving Intercultural Interactions—Implications for the Dance Therapist.* Hunter College, 1996.

This study explores the subject of culture and how it currently applies to the field of mental health and, more specifically, to dance therapy. By recognizing and acknowledging cross cultural differences in a therapeutic relationship, there is less risk that the therapist will misinterpret behaviors of culturally different clients. A first step in being able to communicate on a cross cultural level is understanding culture and what issues inevitably arise out of it. A brief review of the literature on nonverbal communication and cross cultural differences is presented. In order to effectively demonstrate the depth to which culture can effect communication, the author researched the African American culture from cultural, historical and nonverbal perspectives. Issues in having white therapists treat black clients of a lower socioeconomic status were presented including suggestions for improving upon such relationships. A questionnaire was created to identify and assess the awareness and competencies of the dance therapist as they relate to the culturally different. Ten female graduate students, enrolled in the Hunter College Dance/Movement Therapy program, participated in this study. The sampling of students placed high importance on the influence of culture, indicating they were well aware of the importance of becoming culturally skilled.

Durkin, Carmel. *Dance/Movement Therapy: A Psychotherapeutic Process to Support a Child with Emotional and Behavioral Disorder to Cope Effectively Within a Mainstream Classroom.* Laban Centre for Movement and Dance, 1992.

Eaton, Bonnie. *Dancing the Connections, Healing the Splits: Dance Movement Therapy from a Body Oriented Perspective.* Lesley College Graduate School, 1993.

Arguing for a theoretical perspective that encompasses the microcosm and the macrocosm, this paper briefly reviews the theoretical contributions of Reich, Lowen and others in the formulations of body-oriented therapies and uses the Kestenberg Movement Profile to apply these theories to movement/dance therapy. Following the process of self observation through movement, the author examines how splits occur in the body, particularly the splitting off of anger. The author concludes by offering the thoughts of Arthur Egendorf and John P. Conger on the patterns that are universal to the healing process and articulating the way in which the body and its expression through movement is representative of that process.

Eckhaus, Naomi S. *Dance Therapy and Physical Rehabilitation.* Hunter College, 1978.

Recognizing the problem of a lack of psychotherapeutic services in physical rehabilitation, there is a general discussion of the psychological problems that are pertinent to the physically disabled. Specific information is given regarding the physical and psychological aspects of six disabilities commonly found in a rehabilitation center. It is discussed how the physical conditions of each would affect dealing with the psychological conditions through dance therapy. The summary deals with rehabilitation centers generally, and relates the author's experiences in such a center. It concludes that dance therapy may be very valuable in rehabilitation.

Economou, Katerina. *Developing Interaction with an Autistic Child in Dance Movement Therapy.* Laban Centre London, 1996.

This thesis discusses the ways in which dance movement therapy is used to support and increase communication and interaction in children with autism. An understanding of the origins of autism is gained by a comprehensive literature review concerning the biological, physiological, neurological and psychoanalytic factors of autism. A description of twenty dance movement therapy sessions with an autistic child is presented as an illustration of: a) the use of dance movement therapy with a psychoanalytic orientation in autism with psychological determinants, and b) the dance movement techniques and interventions used for stimulating social interaction and developing a relationship with autistic children.

This case study indicates changes in the child's movement qualities and physical activities as well as a significant development of non-verbal communication and interaction. A relationship between the therapist and the child was also formed. The child related to the dance movement therapist as a 'mother' who could eventually provide emotional security. The child showed ability for emotional and physical interaction with the dance movement therapist who physically attuned and reflected the child's behaviour and emotions. An apparent decrease of self-injuring behaviour was reported by the class teacher. Nevertheless, no other behavioural changes were apparent outside the dance movement therapy setting.

Eggerding, Marjorie J. *Numinous Dance Therapy: The Enchanted Dance.* Prescott College, 1994.

This is a study in which it is hypothesized that dance therapy with a specific set of directed dance and movement experiences provides an effective means for developing and/or enhancing spiritual awareness in individuals that have lost this essential human quality of life, particularly those being treated for addictions and/or mental and behavioral disorders in a psychiatric hospital setting.

An overview of the relevant literature pertaining to spiritual, psychological, dance history and dance therapy theories and concepts was presented. Literature describing the spiritually significant aspects of symbol, myth and ritual for dance therapy was also reviewed.

This theoretical and phenomenological study resulted in the development of a theory of spiritually focused dance therapy called Numinous Dance Therapy (NDT). A brief videotaped segment of an NDT session accompanies this thesis along with several journals of participants' spiritual experiences resulting from NDT sessions.

Egido, Elaine M. *A Developmental Perspective on the Use of Dance/Movement Therapy with Adult Children of Alcoholics: A Literature Review.* Allegheny University of the Health Sciences (formerly Hahnemann University), 1991.

This study was undertaken with adult children of alcoholics. The premise is that adult children of alcoholics miss some of the mother/infant interaction which is the foundation of a healthy self image due to the family's focus on alcohol. Dance/movement therapy relies on nonverbal interaction much the same as early interactions of mother/child. Through an overview of early child development and dance/movement therapy literature, a correlation is drawn to ego-forming parenting techniques and interactions, and the parenting components of dance/movement therapy. This is used to support the significance of the use of dance/movement therapy with this population.

El Guindy, Howaida. *The "Zar": Dance Therapy for Egyptian Women.* Hunter College, 1992.

The purpose of this study is to examine one of Egypt's oldest dances, the Zar. This dance is performed for the sole purposes of healing and therapy and is practiced by Moslems, Christians and Jews, in Egypt, the Sudan and Ethiopia where it originated. Dating as far back as the ancient times, the Zar has undergone some minor changes due to the various cultural influences that came through Egypt. Ritual and rhythm remain common aspects in all Zar dances, wherever they are practiced. This paper will present a close look at the Zar's historical and cultural roots, and an analysis of those aspects of the Zar that make it therapeutic. A comparison between the Zar and dance therapy will shed some light on dance therapy's own historical roots. Finally, this paper asks the following questions: what aspects of the Zar can be incorporated in dance therapy, or vice versa, to make both practices more understandable, effective and accessible modalities to the respective populations?

Embers, Jeana. *The Circle of Life Healing Arts Journey.* Antioch/New England Graduate School, 1995.

Creating a theoretical model that integrates Native American Circle of Life concepts with dance-movement therapy and the expressive arts offers clients a way to enhance and further their recovery from dysfunctions, addictions, trauma, etc., along with discovering the relationship of the human being with the planet Earth in order to bring about collective awareness and a means of survival and good health as we move into the Space Age of the twenty-first century.

Native American teachers who walk the medicine way have given the author insight and healing through the Circle of Life. This knowledge, dance/movement therapy concepts, and twenty years of experience with the expressive arts are all being combined to shape this healing arts journey method. Native people traditionally incorporate the arts in their daily lives, and with this awareness, the author offers a format for therapeutic use. Dance, music, art, and drama become the avenues to travel the Circle of Life in order to create balance and wholeness in the center of the sacred hoop of each of our lives. Planetary, human, and animal aspects accentuate the process, with a focus on the physical, emotional, spiritual, and mental attributes of all life.

Errington, Anne. *A Study of Caring and Sharing in Girls from a Roumanian Children's Home.* Laban Centre for Movement and Dance, 1993.

Falk, Marjorie Gail. *Family Therapy and Dance/Movement Therapy: An Integration.* Goucher College, 1993.

The purpose of this thesis, and the resulting educational videotape, is to explore whether the therapeutic process and goals of dance/movement therapy can be used to address family therapy issues. The four issues examined are: the family as a system, subsystem boundaries based on Minuchin's work, communication, and individual differences drawn from Satir's work. This integration is intended to allow clinicians of each discipline to inform and draw from each other.

The literature in family therapy is reviewed and focused on these issues through examining the concepts of the structural (Minuchin) and experiential (Satir) family therapy models, and their respective goals, methods, techniques, therapeutic presence, and use of non-verbal behavior in treatment. The literature in dance/movement therapy is reviewed focusing on groups. Basic principles, goals, methods, techniques, and therapeutic presence are examined. The limited literature on dance/movement therapy with families is reviewed including the areas of family non-verbal interaction studies and parent-child dyads. This information is synthesized with the examination of similarities and points of integration between the two fields.

This integration produced results in the form of a training video. This video depicts the four family therapy issues, which the researcher translated into four movement structures designed to clarify the issue for the family. Graduate students or professionals in the field of dance/movement therapy represented the families. This video also includes an introduction and discussion on the topic of the integration of family and dance/movement therapy.

It concludes that an integration benefits family treatment through providing a rich therapeutic experience and integrating cognitive, emotional, and kinesthetic processes. The videotape visually documents this integration.

Faraone, Caroline J. *The Rise and Fall of University Sponsored Dance Therapy Programs in the United States.* Hunter College, 1996.

Between 1971 and 1984 a total of 19 Dance Therapy programs, both graduate and undergraduate, were opened at public and private universities in the United States. Since 1979, 12 of the 19 programs have closed. Administrative planning, decision making and budget cutting are examined. Key faculty members of six dance therapy programs are interviewed to determine how the roles of visibility, administrative support, enrollment and university politics play in the closing of programs. Implications for the profession and preventative measures are briefly explored.

Farone, Diana. *The Use of Dance/Movement Therapy with Adult Survivors of Sexual Abuse.* University of California, Los Angeles, 1993. (SP)

Farr, Madelyn. *The Role of Dance/Movement Therapy in Treating At-Risk African American Adolescents: A Multicultural Perspective.* Antioch/New England Graduate School, 1995.

Dance/movement therapy (DMT) is presented as a modality of choice in the treatment of at-risk African-American adolescents. Its therapeutic potential is explored from a multicultural perspective that highlights the need for culturally appropriate strategies responsive to the unique psychosocial challenges facing these youths. The role of dance in Black America, from its tribal roots to the streets of urban centers, establishes a precedent for its proposed function as a restorative agent. The affective and relational features of Black behaviors are considered to support the advantages of DMT in accommodating characteristic cultural styles. Cross-cultural issues in the treatment of at-risk Black youths are integrated in a formulation of a DMT theory and method. An experiential application of DMT techniques is described in this writer's account of her work with the population, supported by case examples to illustrate the modality's treatment value. It is argued that DMT can effectively engage the creativity and resilience inherent in this population's coping repertoire towards greater adaptive and growthful functioning.

Fear, Leslie. *DMT with Hospitalized Children in a Child Life Program.* Hunter College, 1994.

This paper is the study of the integration of dance/movement therapy into a child life program serving hospitalized children. Many guiding principles of both disciplines were found to be similar.

Federman, Dita. *Dance Movement Therapy Groups with Personality Disturbed In-Patients—An Integrative Model.* Lesley College Graduate School, 1992.

In recent years, patients with personality disorders have become a focus of interest for mental health professionals. Since disturbances in interpersonal relationships are a hallmark of this population, group psychotherapy can offer a valuable therapeutic method in treating patients with these disorders. Low self image is common among this population, and since body image is part of self-image, dance movement therapy groups have become of significant importance.

This study is designed to present an integrative model for treatment of personality disorder patients. Different structural group models integrating verbal and nonverbal processes and their potential to bring about an improvement in interpersonal relationships, intimacy and self-image of personality disorder patients are presented.

Few, Joseph Bocage. *Dance Therapy Theater: An Exploration of Creativity and Community Toward Education.* Naropa Institute, 1991.

Fischbach, Monica. *Movement Indicators in The Kestenberg Movement Profile as an Assessment Tool in Posttraumatic Stress Disorder Resulting From Physical or Sexual Abuse.* Antioch/New England Graduate Program, 1996.

The purpose of this thesis is to show how the concepts of the Kestenberg Movement Profile can provide movement indicators for the diagnosis and evaluation of Posttraumatic Stress Disorder resulting from sexual or physical abuse. Based on the data derived from the observation of several known survivors, certain movement qualities were seen that could be interpreted to indicate that abuse occurred. Movement factors in the KMP also seem to indicate preferred methods of coping and defense. Together, all the information obtained either from movement observations or from notation using the KMP, can provide a valuable tool both in assessment and in the formulation of treatment.

Fishbein, Tema. *The Development of Body Image, It's Clinical Implications in Dance/Movement Therapy: A Case Study.* Hunter College, 1985.

This study explores the development of body image from infancy to early childhood, reviewing developmental theorists and researchers to define the variables in the environment which influences and shapes human development. A case study is presented describing dance/movement therapy with a child who has severe body image disturbance. The author recreates the therapeutic process of meeting the client at the stage of her developmental arrest, and helping her to travel the path to a healthy image of her body. The case study examines the child's developmental arrest, how it was diagnosed, and confirms the usefulness of dance/movement therapy in reconstructing a body image which was functional and appropriate to the child's age.

Fledderjohn, Heidi and Sewickley, Judith. *An Annotated Bibliography of Dance/Movement Therapy: 1940-1990.* Goucher College, 1991.

The purpose of this project is to create an annotated bibliography of published clinical and theoretical literature in the field of dance/movement therapy. The methodology is divided into three phases: 1) searching and gathering, 2) securing and annotating source material, 3) integrating and restructuring according to the literature. Source material for the bibliography was gathered from a variety of sources. Manual and computer searches accessed the following areas of study: arts and humanities, education, medicine, psychology and social sciences. The final project is divided into two sections; theoretical and research material in dance/movement therapy and clinical practice in dance/movement therapy. The theoretical chapter includes information addressing the philosophies and doctrines of dance/movement therapy. The clinical practice section contains the following subchapters: Adolescent Disorders, Anxiety Disorders, Childhood Disorders, Eating Disorders, Family, Geriatrics, Mood Disorders, Neuroses, Personality Disorders, Physical and Sexual Abuse, Schizophrenia, Somatic Disorders, Substance Abuse and Traumatic Brain Injury.

Fleischer, Karin. *The Bridge: A Comparative Analysis of Selected Disciplines on the Impact of the Transcendent Experience on Conscious Personality.* California State University, Hayward, 1994.

This is a comparative study on the integration of the personal and the transpersonal realm. The focus is on the impact of a transcendent experience on the individual's conscious personality. The first two stages of a spiritual initiation process are described from the perspective of the following disciplines: authentic movement, depth psychology, Christian mysticism, shamanism and Hinduism.

Foglietti, Rebecca. *Dance/Movement Therapy and Hope in People Living with AIDS.* Naropa Institute, 1995.

In the past two decades research increasingly points to a connection between emotional states and physical health. Feelings such as hope are believed not only to extend life span, but to improve quality of life. The importance of integration between bodily felt sensation and emotional/mental states is a core tenant in dance/movement therapy. Awareness of physical sensation can lead to expression of emotion, which may be empowering. This process can reconnect people with a sense of hope, or strengthen that which is already present. People living with AIDS comprise a population in which hope is both essential and yet also challenging. They present an opportunity to examine the potential effects of dance/movement therapy on hope. Hypothesis: Dance/movement therapy can significantly increase hope in people living with AIDS. Four male and one female subject were administered the Herth Hope Scale before and after completing four sessions of dance/movement therapy. Intervention focused on awareness, expression, and empowerment. Data was analyzed by direct difference, correlated t-test. Overall scores and 2 of 3 factors showed no significant change. Factor U, Positive Readiness & Expectancy, showed a significant increase at the .05 level of confidence. Difficulties with study design and outcome are discussed as well as implications for further research.

Fountaine, Lois H. *Perspectives on Afro-American Culture and Nonverbal Communications.* Hunter College, 1982.

This paper explores the culture and nonverbal communications of Afro-Americans. The effects of slavery, racism and racial theories and how these factors have influenced Afro-American culture are examined. The importance for dance therapists to understand Afro-American culture as a referent for observing and interpreting their nonverbal communication is also discussed.

Fowler, Brandi Beck. *The Importance of Empathy for Eating Disordered Patients: Dance/Movement Therapy and the Relational Model.* Antioch/New England Graduate School, 1996.

This thesis explores the process which five Southern African adolescent girls who suffered from anorexia worked through in their quest to rebuild a sense of self, experience empathy and develop a greater sense of freedom towards their bodies within the framework of dance movement therapy. The young women in these case studies come from different ethnic backgrounds of Southern Africa. This played a part in their diagnosis of anorexia and had a visible effect on the dance movement therapy group being discussed. This thesis focuses on the process each young woman went through in embracing certain archetypes while trying to establish empathy and recreate more flexible self boundaries. The self-in-relation theory will be addressed as it was used in the dance/movement therapy group. Close examination of the process focuses on their growing trust in both the therapist and their own bodies, and their ability to become empathic towards each other and themselves. The use of archetypes evolved out of their immediate resistance to movement and from the therapist's attempt to provide a new creative medium of expression and identification. The goal of the therapist was to encourage exploration of their own bodies, self boundaries, and identities while providing them with a safe container and an interesting medium. Clinical case studies have been included as they relate to the use of Jungian archetype as a metaphor for creative movement exploration and the patient/client's development of a new movement vocabulary. These studies address the patients' development of a healthier body image that was transformed through dance movement therapy techniques. By recognizing both their ability to empathize and their need for relationships, the patients were able to progress beyond their previous boundaries. A brief history of the ethnic origin of each girl has been included.

Fraenkel, Danielle L. *The Inns and Outs of Medical Excounters: An Interactional Analysis of Empathy, Patient Satisfaction, and Information Exchange.*
University of Rochester, 1986. (C-Doctoral)

This study integrated concepts from medicine, counseling and dance therapy to explore the relationships among varying levels of empathy, dyadic nonverbal behaviors, patient satisfaction, and patient recall of doctor-offered information. The researcher examined the relationship of the physicians's sex to these variables. Three concepts provided the foundation for the study: 1) Barrett-Lennard's interactional, clinical , and phenomenological analysis of empathy; 2) synchrony and echoing—units of interactional analysis—used to summarize the physician's and patient's nonverbal interactions; 3) Kagan's Interpersonal Process Recall System (IPRS) used to tap the moment-to-moment changing perceptions of the physicians level of empathy.

Twelve male and seven family medicine residents and 19 of their female patients were videotaped during the pre-physical and post-physical segments of their encounters. After the appointment, the subject used the IPRS to label perceptions of physician's level of empathy, completed a state satisfaction questionnaire, and described recall of what doctor had said. One group of raters scored the tapes with audio off for synchrony and echoing; a second group rated audio only for doctor-offered information. The two analyses were combined to identify the information accompanied by synchrony and echoing.

While total echoing, total synchrony, and the total echoing accompanying information-giving failed to relate to empathy, satisfaction, or recall, integrants of echoing and synchrony generated relationships with empathy and accurate recall, respectively, which merit further examination. Total empathy correlated moderately with satisfaction; affective and cognitive empathy alone did not. Affective empathy correlated moderately with information-giving regarding the patient's treatment and regimen.

New ways of thinking about synchrony, echoing, empathy and patient recall were presented: the consideration of patient initiated echoing as a marker for affective process; doctor initiated echoing as a marker for cognitive process; synchrony as a kinesthetic signal for accurate recall; a change in empathy training curricula; and support for the view of empathy as multidimensional. The methodological and technical limitations of the study and suggestions for using synchrony and echoing to analyze dyadic and group settings in medicine, education and counseling/psychotherapy were discussed.

Franken, Forest. *The Value of Dance/Movement Therapy in Working with Cancer Patients.* University of California, Los Angeles, 1995. (SP)

Frant, Phyllis. *Dynamic Therapy for the Aphasic Patient.* Hunter College, 1972.
An overview of the aphasic individual and it implications for dance therapy.

Fucius, Yulan. *Into The Storm: Dance/Movement Therapy as a Primary Clinical Treatment With Conduct Disorder.* Antioch/New England Graduate School, 1991.
Dance/movement therapy is presented as the primary clinical treatment modality for Adolescent Conduct Disorder. Leading to this postulation is background information concerning the evolution in parental and social attitude relating to adolescence, the understanding of normal adolescent development stage, and the information on the etiology, diagnosis and treatment issues of Adolescent Conduct Disorder. Also discussed are the deficits in the existing treatment systems and a comparison between conventional therapy approach and dance/movement therapy. This comparison illuminates the essential employment of dance/movement therapy for treatment of Conduct Disorder.

The three major treatment issues discussed are affect/behavioral modulation, interaction/socialization, and developmental tasks for the formation of age-appropriate ego-self as well as sexual identity. Treatment issues and goals are discussed with reference to mainstream psychotherapy rationale and to Dance Therapy clinical grounding. Recommendations are appended for the differentiation and integration of role images as a Dance Psychotherapist for effective intervention with adolescents having Conduct Disorder.

Funderburk, Judith B. *Healing the Whole Person: A Process-Oriented Expressive Arts Approach to Therapy.* Vermont College of Norwich University, 1992. (Available from author: jvictor@erols.com)
A synthesis of process-oriented approaches to healing from ancient to modern times is presented in this thesis. Perennial philosophy, shamanic healing arts, the Life/Art Process of Anna Halprin, expressive arts (especially dance/movement) therapy, and aspects of the work of Carl Jung, Fritz Perls, Arnold Mindell and Ken Wilber are examined. The applicability of a process-oriented expressive arts approach as a treatment for persons with eating disorders is demonstrated. The author's personal process are included as a related case study describing beginning recovery from bulimia. Artwork and descriptions of expressive movement sequences are incorporated. Recommendations are made for implementation of this process-oriented expressive arts approach to healing in light of new discoveries about the mind/body connection. Included is extensive list of references and an annotated bibliography.

Gary, Gomer. *Holistic Practice In Mental Health.* Hunter College, 1981.
A report on the Dual Degree Program in Dance Therapy and Social Work.

Gaudreau, Ruth. *Creating a Temenos For Menarche Using Dance Movement Therapy.* Antioch/New England Graduate School, 1995.
The purpose of this thesis is to create a celebration as a way of marking a young girl's passage into

physical womanhood. The focus here is on prevention of negative body images and attitudes about menses and womanhood. The emphasis is on pro-action of the development of young women's sense of self in an appropriate and safe environment. A cross-culture literature review on the history of menarche rituals or female pubertal rites of passage and a literature review on menarche rituals in dance/movement therapy are examined. This thesis addressed the importance of female pubertal rites of passage and how dance/movement therapists can facilitate acknowledgment of this important milestone. A proposed designed celebration, tools and techniques are suggested as a way of providing this service to young women.

Geller, Janice. *The Integrative Therapy Model of Self: An Interdisciplinary Approach to Resolving Early Object Relations Issues.* California State University, Hayward, 1994.

A theoretical exploration of psychological development and how the retrieval of memories are accessed through the body and movement. A personal exploration developed the integrative therapy model.

Gellman, Leigh. *The Influence of Dance/Movement Intervention on the Development of Normal Preschoolers.* Allegheny University of the Health Sciences (formerly Hahnemann University), 1995.

This study examines the influence of a dance/movement intervention on the development of normal preschoolers. It attempts to provide empirical data on the effect of dance/movement intervention on child development. Twenty-four subjects from a private Philadelphia preschool were involved in the study. The subjects received a pre-test using the Developmental Profile II, a standardized measure of child development with sub-scales for five major areas of development. The subjects were then divided into experimental groups either receiving dance/movement intervention, or attention control groups, which received no dance/movement intervention but an equivalent time with an art activity. The intervention was for a 30 minutes weekly for thirteen weeks. Upon completion of the thirteen weeks, a post-test of the Developmental Profile II was administered to all subjects. This study was based on the hypothesis that the subjects receiving the dance/movement intervention will show greater differences between pre-test and post-test scores on the Developmental Profile II than those children who do not. The findings of this study supported this hypothesis. The experimental group demonstrated a highly significant difference from pre-test to post-test on the physical developmental scale. The other areas of development as measured by Developmental Profile II showed no significant change. Significance of the results and implications are explored.

Giannone, Gina Marie. *Moving up with Downs: A Dance Movement Therapist's Perspective on Enhancing Socialization with Down Syndrome Adolescents.* Hunter College, 1993.

Ginga, Marie. *Moving Towards Health: Dance/Movement Therapy and Physical Healing.* Antioch/New England Graduate School, 1996.

This thesis explores how dance/movement therapy can be helpful in supporting physical healing. It is a useful guide to all professionals in health related fields who wish to expand their understanding of the healing process. Briefly exploring the history of mind/body medicine, it presents in more detail contemporary thoughts and theories about how the mind and the body work together towards healing. It includes work currently being done by dance therapists in this field and explores in depth a program designed by Dr. Bernie Siegel called Exceptional Cancer Patients (ECaP) that uses psychological healing to support allopathic medicine. Dance/movement therapy complements this process both in theory and techniques. A program is developed that works within the parameters and guidelines of Dr. Siegel's work. There is a summary of both programs and discusses future work in this area.

Glenn, Marlene. *Video Tape Analysis Concerning Issues of Separation-Individuation.* Hunter College, 1991.

A dance therapy session on a short term unit was videotaped in order to study how a therapist handles issues of separation-individuation in a dance therapy group. Chosen parameters reveal the therapist's need for attachment. Therapist's reactions to separation issues have a major effect on the outcome of the session.

Glenski, Robin. *Socio/Dance Therapy: An Innovative Response to a Financial Crunch.* Antioch/New England Graduate School, 1993.

Limited funding within the institutional environment often inhibits the growth and development of dance therapy as a distinct therapeutic modality. While mental health facilities may be willing to hire a single or "token" dance therapist, budgetary constraints often make it a challenge to add positions and create a dance therapy department. This paper focuses on this dilemma and an innovative response to the challenge: the creation of a new job position, Socio/Dance Therapy. Socio/Dance Therapy is a conglomerate of two modes of clinical intervention, sociotherapy and dance therapy. The author describes her unusual perspective from her position as a sociotherapist and as a dance therapy intern on the same treatment team.

Goehring, C. Griffin. *Activity and Passivity: A Movement Metaphor For Control and Surrender in Early Recovery From Addictions.* Antioch/New England Graduate School, 1993.

This thesis examines the use of dance/movement therapy with persons participating in short term in-patient treatment for recovery from chemical addictions. A primary task of this early stage of healing is learning to surrender one's struggle to exert control over the addictive substance while learning to take responsible action towards sobriety. Creative dance material exploring the polarities of activity and passivity was used to create an embodied experience of this paradox inherent in the recovery process. Clinical vignettes describe the application of the dance material to treatment goals, which are organized around the Twelve Step Program of Alcoholics Anonymous.

Goldman, Deborah Rae. *Reclaiming the Dark Goddess: Dances in the Collective Unconscious.* Lesley College Graduate School, 1996.

The purpose of this study is to explore the archetypal image of the Dark Goddess in order to reclaim what has been repressed in the collective unconscious. It proposes that by cutting off the power of the Goddess, our culture has repressed the wisdom of bodily experience; aspects of our sexuality, power, spirituality, authenticity, and vulnerability. The Great Goddess is explored as a paradigm for understanding the human experience; as a process of life, death, and regeneration; and as an archetypal image. It does this by 1) presenting a feminist revisioning of archetypal psychology, 2) examining the mythology of the Great Goddess, 3) looking at how this Goddess has been repressed in a culture which has shifted to a paradigm of linear dualism, 4) presenting the Goddess as a powerful, unified archetypal image for healing a fragmented culture and a fragmented self, 6) and grounding this work in Expressive Therapy, particularly Dance/Movement Therapy.

Aspects of heuristic, historical, and creative process methodologies have been combined in addressing the above objectives. This thesis relates to the fields of expressive therapy, dance/movement therapy, and psychology. It is also relevant to those seeking wholeness through an understanding of the sacredness of their own body.

Goldman, Lisa. *Dance/Movement Therapy and the Brain-Injured Client: The Empathic Connection.* Columbia College, 1996.

This thesis is about survivors of traumatic brain injury. It is an exploration of the emotional challenges that these survivors experience as they reintegrate into society. In response to their brain injury these persons are challenged with physical, cognitive, and emotional deficits. They are "different" than they were prior to their injury. This thesis looks at how to assist the survivor of brain injury, through the use of dance/movement therapy, in becoming empathic toward their own process of healing. It makes use of Marian Chace's four core concepts of dance/movement therapy and her empathic reflection theory which focuses on the creation of the empathic environment. This empathic environment serves as a fundamental precursor to the process of self integration. There is a discussion of how dance/movement therapy, as a body-centered therapy which involves a release of tension, further facilitates this integration of the self. The release of tension, specifically with the survivor of traumatic brain injury, enables the client to experience emotional as well as physical relief. This study provides an in depth understanding of the role of dance/movement therapy in the recovery and reintegration process of the survivor of brain injury through information, clinical observations and the discussion of one case study to illuminate the effectiveness of dance/movement therapy with this population.

Goldman-Nevins, Karen Lee. *The Observation and Analysis of Kinesthetic Empathy in the Dance/Movement Therapy Encounter.* Allegheny University of the Health Sciences (formerly Hahnemann University), 1993.

The purpose of this thesis is to develop refined criteria for describing the way that kinesthetic empathy occurs in the dance/movement therapy context. When the body is used to facilitate empathic understanding it is called kinesthetic empathy. Empathy is important for the establishment of an effective patient-therapist relationship. This research provides detailed parameters for evaluating the presence and quality of empathy within the dance/movement therapy context. Techniques are described for identifying the empathic process and a discussion is provided on the risks of using the body to facilitate empathy. The research specifically tests a pilot scale for observing and recording elements of kinesthetic empathy, based upon three dyadic dance/movement therapy interactions which were videotaped by three trained observers. Results include data on inter-observer agreement, and on empathy-related aspects of the dance/movement therapy interaction. A review of theorists' definitions of empathy, the use of empathy in traditional psychotherapy and the way that empathy is manifested in the dance/movement therapy context frames the presentation.

Goldsand, R.A. *Dance/Movement Therapy as Treatment Modality for Sexually Abused Children: Two Case Studies.* Hunter College, 1985.

The purpose of this study is to examine the efficacy of dance/movement therapy with sexually abused children. The philosophies and opinions of professionals in the fields of child development, sexual abuse, and dance/movement therapy are presented. Two case studies are provided in order to illustrate dance/movement therapy treatment with two emotionally disturbed children (a boy aged 9 and a girl aged 12) who have been sexually abused by their respective opposite-sex parents. This includes: history and background information, movement preferences and tendencies, goals and themes which evolved over the course of treatment and finally an analysis. It is concluded that dance/movement therapy is an effective treatment modality for sexually abused children.

Goldschlag-Teich, Miri. *Jazz Dance with Adolescents as a Means of Therapeutic Change.* Lesley College Graduate School, 1995.

Jazz dance is reviewed from its beginnings in the African savanna. The development of this peculiar music and dance style being closely related to American history mirrors the development of culture and ethnic arts in this part of the world. Further inspiration from this music style has influenced the conservative classic dance, giving birth to new dance styles eventually contributing to principles of movement therapy as well.

The classic psychological bases and principles are detailed. Problems faced by adolescents as individuals or in groups are analyzed from different points of view. A jazz dance group of adolescent girls has been surveyed for two years. They answered a questionnaire that tried to define the therapeutic process. Four individual cases are described together with conclusions about the group.

Goldstein, Lisa I. *Sign of the Self/Heredity of The Self: A Case Study Using The Kestenberg Movement Profile in Dance/Movement Therapy With a Learning Disabled Child With a Focus on Learning Styles.* Antioch/New England Graduate School, 1996.

The purpose of this case study is to investigate how dance/movement therapy is used to help a child with difficulty communicating. Emotional blocks are investigated for how they block learning styles. Also explored are how the emotional components associated with alternative learning styles are expressed and manifested. The dance/movement therapy process and the methods used to help the child are examined and recorded. Highlighted in this study is the use of the Kestenberg Movement Profile to discover the subjects learning styles and emotional blocks to learning. It is revealed how dance/movement therapy helped in the process of developing skills for successful learning. The therapy process is guided by existing clinical and educational treatment goals and assessments with dance/movement therapy as the treatment vehicle. As part of the case study a video was taken. The movements of the child were analyzed using parts of the Kestenberg Movement Profile.

Gonnella, Nicole. *Dance/Movement Therapy with a Children's Group: A Comparison Analysis of Group Process.* Allegheny University of the Health Sciences (formerly Hahnemann University), 1996.

Dance/movement therapy (d/mt) often includes therapeutic practice with groups of children. However the d/mt literature is silent on the specific topic of group dynamics in d/mt groups for children. This study was devised to observe children in a d/mt group. It examines the assessments of two children's groups made by two different pairs of professionals. The researcher expected that the two different analyses of the groups would be similar. The children ranged in age from six to nine and were grouped according to gender. One session of each group's weekly d/mt group was video taped for analysis. Two dance/movement therapists (D/MTs) and two group therapists (Gps) observed the video tapes of each group to assess the developmental level of the groups according to Bennis and Shepherd's theory of group development. The two pairs of professionals agreed on the developmental phase of the girl's group, while the D/MTs and one of the Gps agreed on the boy's group. The results support the expectations of the study. The data implies that d/mt may not only use movement observation to form group assessment. It is suggested in order to fully understand children in groups, a study be designed to devise a theory for group development in children.

Gonzales, Paula S. *Dance Therapy and Autism: A Case Study of Miss J.* Hunter College, 1994.

This case study focuses on the therapeutic relationship between the author and a predominantly nonverbal, autistic three year old child. The behaviors common to autistic children are identified and educational, behavioral and psychoanalytic treatment approaches are reviewed. The author focuses on several methods used within each approach, specifically mainstreaming behavior modification, humanistic education, and the Linwood method to augment the dance therapy interventions.

Gonzalez, Carla Antonia. *Dance/Movement Therapy with Childhood Post-Traumatic Stress Disorder.* Goucher College, 1993.

This thesis is designed to explore the therapeutic goals, methods, and techniques that are consistently successful, as reported by registered dance/movement therapists, for the treatment of childhood post-traumatic stress disorder (PTSD). The author interviewed five registered dance/movement therapists who have past experience or who are currently working with this population to discover the goals, methods, and techniques they find successful for the treatment of childhood PTSD. A review of the literature on childhood PTSD, dance/movement therapy, and previous research relevant to both is presented.

Conclusions of this study indicate that for this population, movement serves as a channel through which relationships can be formed or repaired with peers and adults, thus diminishing pathological anxiety. The primary therapeutic goals are forming a therapeutic alliance, enhancing self awareness and body awareness, and increasing self-esteem. The dance/movement therapists aid the child in accomplishing these goals by validating, labeling, modeling, and identifying feelings and behaviors, expanding breath and range of movement, providing clear structures and limits, and assisting the child in mastering the environment. These conclusions are presented in five case studies. The similarities between the interviewees' answers and the significance of these are discussed.

Goss, Heather Colleen. *Concepts and Methods of Dance/Movement Therapy in Working with Eating Disorders.* Goucher College, 1992.

This study is an examination of eating disorders, specifically anorexia and bulimia, in order to conceptualize dance/movement therapy treatment with this population. A literature review of eating disorders provides definitions, diagnostic criteria and includes the history, etiology and treatment approaches of the eating disorder population.

A review of dance/movement therapy literature comprises the history of dance/movement therapy through ritual dances and healing and the contributions of dance/movement therapy pioneers to the field. Principles, goals, process, interventions and techniques of dance/movement therapy are outlined and then examined in relation to an eating disorder population.

Ten dance/movement therapists who have worked with this population were interviewed for this study. The therapists were asked questions regarding background information, training, work settings and experience with an eating disorder population. Questions were asked regarding theoretical orientation, classification system, effectiveness of dance/movement therapy and how dance/movement therapy is utilized with an eating disorder population.

Issues, goals, methods and techniques for anorexics and bulimics were extrapolated from the interviews. A conceptual framework consisting of treatment programs, characteristics, issues and themes, goals, techniques, treatment process and special considerations was formulated. The results of this study indicate that dance/movement therapy is useful in working with an eating disorder population.

Gorscak, Kathleen J. *The Study of Proxemics with Synchrony and ADHD Symptoms in a Movement Session with Attention Deficit Hyperactive Children.* Hunter College, 1992.

This study examines the relationship of proxemics with synchrony and the symptoms of ADHD featured children in a movement session. The hypothesis of the study states that when proxemic boundaries are altered for ADHD children, there is an increase in the amount of synchrony. As a result of increased synchrony, there is a decrease in ADHD symptoms. The symptoms of ADHD children are hyperactivity, impulsivity, and inattention.

In a movement session, ADHD children need structure, consistency, and containment. A videotape of a movement session with ADHD children was observed for three minute segments by trained raters. In each segment the children were seated in different arrangements, allowing for closer proximity by the last segment. The raters observed synchronous movement and ADHD symptoms. The results of the study show low scores in synchronous movement and decreased scores in ADHD symptoms as the proxemics became closer. Therefore, it was found that synchronous movement did not correlate with close proxemics or with ADHD symptoms. However, the results do show a correlation that when proxemics are closer, ADHD symptoms decrease.

Gowen, Gerald. *A Theoretical Integration of Dasein Analysis and Dance/Movement Therapy.* Allegheny University of the Health Sciences (formerly Hahnemann University), 1991.

This study was undertaken in attempt to integrate the dance/movement therapy approach with the existential, phenomenological and ontological approach of Dasein analytic psychotherapy. It was hypothesized that Effort/Shape theory provides an ideal existential and phenomenological way to understand each person's possibilities for being open and receptive to Being-in-the-world with one's own being, others and the world, and ultimately in relation to Being. It was also hypothesized that movement and creativity are both primary and significant in revealing a person's existential nature as a bundle of possibilities for being deeply related to Being. The paper is a literature review focused primarily on the integration of Dasein analysis, related phenomenology, relevant existentialism, pertinent Jungian psychology, hypnosis and trance phenomena, and dance/movement therapy and creativity. A daseinanalytic dance/movement therapy approach is developed and outlined. "Being-with" was explored in a one hour video taped session with four subjects. In conclusion, the thesis integrated the above literature sources and developed several new concepts regarding the mechanisms by which we experience metaphor, symbols and archetypes through dance/movement. It is suggested that in therapy, creative intelligence may be a person's ability to attune to the Effort rhythms shared between Self, other, world, and Being and that creative intelligence may be correlated with Laban's Inner States.

Gray, Shauna. *"Dance/Movement Therapy: Yes It's All Very Nice, But Does It Work?"* Antioch/New England Graduate School 1995.

This thesis examines the impact two multi-disciplinary outpatient chronic pain treatment programs have on two participants over their 12 week treatment period. Participant B participated in dance/movement therapy in conjunction with daily treatment. Participant A received no dance/movement therapy with treatment. A pre- and post-test method of testing, using portions of the Kestenberg Movement Profile, are utilized. A discussion of the comparative findings are presented, as well as implications this study has for the field of dance/movement therapy.

Green, Nona Michelle. *Dance/Movement Therapy with Emotionally Handicapped Adolescents in More and Less Restrictive Environments.* Goucher College, 1993.

The purpose of this study is to examine the use of dance/ movement therapy with emotionally handicapped (EH) adolescent males (11-16) exhibiting conduct, mood, and anxiety disorders in residential treatment centers, and to formulate implications of the findings for the use of dance/ movement therapy with this population in less restrictive settings. There are six intensities of special education services (I-VI) available to handicapped children. The approach of this study is designed so that observations made in a the most restrictive setting, a long term residential treatment center, (V-VI) can be utilized to justify the use of dance/movement therapy methods in less restrictive environments (I-IV) where treatment is primarily focused on educational needs of the children. Theories of adolescent development, normal difficulties of adolescence, common psychopathology, and treatment goals are presented. The six levels of special education services are described. Similarities in psychiatric diagnosis and treatment goals for adolescents at these levels will be indicated. Dance/ movement therapy and its definition, history, principles, skills, process, and goals are explained and the literature on dance/movement therapy with EH adolescent males is reviewed. Clinical documentation centered on identified problem behaviors is compiled from medical records and ongoing dance/movement therapy with EH adolescents in an area residential treatment center.

Through the integration of literature and data on adolescence, special education, and dance/ movement therapy it is concluded that EH adolescents in special education (Intensities l-IV) could benefit from dance/movement therapy interventions. Connections between the problems/needs of this population, the goals of dance/movement therapy, and the function/structure of the special education system were drawn. The results provide support for the incorporation of dance/movement therapy into the special education system.

Greenberg, Ruth. *Touch and Verbalization in Four Dance Therapy Sessions.* Hunter College, 1985.

This study's hypothesis is that when touch occurs in a dance therapy session, the amount of verbalization increases; therefore an increase in touch will result in an increase in verbalization. Four dance therapy sessions with psycho-geriatric outpatients were videotaped and analyzed (two sessions with touch and two sessions without touch). Five minutes at the beginning, five minutes in the middle, and five minutes at the end in each of the four video taped dance therapy sessions were randomly chosen to be observed by two raters. The two raters recorded the number of times they observed touch and verbalization occur. It appeared that there was no significant difference in the number of verbalizations in the two sessions with touch, versus the two sessions without touch. It appeared that this group and its leader was limited in its ability to explore feelings through verbalization, and expression of emotional content was improved through the use of touch.

Greenberg, Wendy. *A Phenomenological Study of the Use of Symbolism in Dance Therapy.* Hunter College, 1982.

A structural analysis of the movements and verbalizations contained in a group dance therapy session, identifying the function and form of symbolism in dance therapy. Major aspects included in this study are: how the symbol arises, its form and appearance, how it is used, its relationship to verbal imagery and its therapeutic effect on the group.

Greene, Sajit W. *Play and Cohesion in Adult Dance/Movement Therapy Groups in the Acute Inpatient Setting.* Naropa Institute, 1994.

This thesis investigates the effect of play on group cohesiveness in dance/movement therapy sessions with adult psychiatric inpatients in acute treatment. Group cohesion is considered an important therapeutic factor, and the theories and methods of group dance/movement therapy are oriented toward facilitating interaction and bonding between group members, yet the development of cohesion may be challenged by many factors of the acute, inpatient setting. This study hypothesizes that play enhances group cohesiveness.

This descriptive study presents and discusses five case vignettes in order to correlate occurrences of play and changing levels of group cohesion. These vignettes describe single-session dance/movement therapy groups that took place on the psychiatric unit of a general hospital. Narrative descriptions of each case are accompanied by the results of a cohesiveness measure. The results are also shown in graphic form.

The results of this study indicate that play does enhance the development of group cohesion in dance/movement therapy sessions with adult, psychiatric inpatients. The influence of factors such as types of play, characteristics of group members, and group dynamics are also discussed. This study also includes a review of the dance/movement therapy, group psychotherapy, and play literature, as well as suggestions for further studies.

Gronlund, Erna. *Children's Emotions Processed in Dance: Dance Therapy for Children with Early Emotional Disturbances.* University of Stockholm, Dept. of Pedagogics and University College of Dance, Stockholm, 1994. (Doctoral - Swedish with 12 page English summary).

This dissertation describes dance therapy for children with early emotional disturbances. It is based on five years of experimental work with dance therapy for six children with deep emotional disturbances and serious contact problems.

The process of dance therapy is studied by means of a detailed case study documenting the development of an eight-year old autistic boy in terms of capacity for contact, body image, conflict processing, emotions and object relations. Within the case study the method of dance therapy is analyzed. Patterns are sought throughout the study group and results reported for the entire group as to why did changes occur and can one identify the turning points that changed the direction of the process and contributed to change? What proved effective?

Various methods of data collection and registration are used, primarily qualitative methods. The process of dance therapy is studied with the help of a combination of direct and participant observation plus video obsservations. The children's parents, teachers and therapists and four of the six children were interviewed. In order to counteract subjectivity in the study, consulting judges were employed to check evaluations of development and results. Various assessments of development were made at the start of dance therapy in order to get a baseline from which results could be tested.

Object relation theory is used for explaining how the child in dance therapy is developing his capacity to relate. At the start, all the children were at a low level of object relations and at the end they had all reached a higher level. Dance therapy proved successful since by simultaneously processing both body and emotion, it had twice the effect.

Gross, Carola. *Body Image Concept in Dance Movement Therapy.* Laban Centre for Movement and Dance, 1992.

Guffy, Judy. *The Use of Dance/Movement Therapy with a Correctional Prison Population.* University of California, Los Angeles, 1995. (SP)

Guthrie, Jane. *Evaluation of a Movement and Dance Therapy Program in Head Injury Rehabilitation.* University of Melbourne, 1996. (Available Education Resource Centre, Univ. of Melbourne, Parkville, 3052 Australia).

The thesis reports on the application of Movement and Dance Therapy (MDT) in head injury rehabilitation. The research adopted a mixed method approach to examine whether a cause and effect relationship could be established between MDT and movement quality and control. Sub-categories of questions posed related to whether MDT could increase movement range, adaptability to the environment, postural awareness and alignment, and movement confidence.

The research design and details were decided by clinical circumstances. The study, largely empirical, also involved movement observation and subject report via documentation and interview. The major procedure was an ABA single case design. A balance of quantitative and qualitative procedures were employed including videotape time sampling of movement behavior over nine weeks in the case design; comparisons of the subject within MDT over time; the subject's own perceptions of change; and a time and task analysis of selected outcomes.

The research results indicated that MDT contributed to changes that occurred. The graphic displays of ABA case results demonstrated a majority of plateau or near plateau baseline situations and definite responses to treatment. This outcome was supported by the results of the additional procedures.

Although the sample size prevents generalization of the results to the head injury population, the reseearcher suggests that a cause and effect relationship betwen MDT and the research outcomes was established. The research endeavoured to build a bridge between physiotherapy and MDT, advocating the use of the movement assessment tool, Laban Movement Analysis, in physiotherapy and MDT rehabilitation.

Hale, Leanna S. *Moving Through Birth: Analysis and Implications of Pre- and Perinatal Movement Patterns that Surface in Holotropic Breathwork.* Naropa Institute, 1995.

This work aims at identifying various patterns of movement, breath and body activity as they relate to in-depth psychological work dealing with material from the realm of pre- and perinatal experience, Divisions of pre- and perinatal experience will be based on Stanislav Grof's model of Holotropic Breathwork. In this model the perinatal realm is identified by four basic perinatal matrices (BPM I-IV), each of which have defined psychological features associated with the experience. The author investigates these patterns as they relate to these four pre- and perinatal experiences.

The strategy for this study involves a comprehensive review of existing literature that pertains to Holotropic Breathwork, pre- and perinatal experiences, and Christine Caldwell's somatic therapy that is geared toward facilitating pre- and perinatal issues. An investigation of patterns was conducted by submitting a Survey of MovementObservations to participating certified practitioners of Holotropic Breathwork. Data from this survey was analyzed to reveal typical patterns of movement, breath and body activity as they relate to the experiences of the four BMPs.

The goal of this study is to reveal patterns of movement, breath and body activity as they relate to the unique experiences of each BPM providing therapists with a somatic understanding of pre-and perinatal experience. It is also hoped that the knowledge presented in Caldwell's model of working with these issues may provide practitioners of Holotropic Breathwork with a deeper understanding of the possibilities for facilitating pre- and perinatal issues.

Hallmark, Elizabeth. *Toward Integration: DMT in Cultural Context.* Antioch/ New England Graduate School, 1990.

This thesis presents the view that dance/movement therapy and its professional organization, the American Dance Therapy Association (ADTA), are clear reflections of modern culture's dichotomy between the unconscious and consciousness. To this end, the author examines the body/mind split so prevalent in our culture, and how dance movement therapy developed to address this separation. The thesis traces how the professional identities of dance movement therapists evolved between the first and second generation of practitioners, and explores how socioeconomic factors, the feminist movement of the 1960s, and the establishment of the ADTA contributed to those identity changes. Primarily framing her ideas with Jungian theory, the author shows that the profession had its beginnings within unconscious creative process and that the profession has now shifted toward a current emphasis on public identity and organization. These two polarities in the field of dance/ movement therapy parallel the cultural body/mind split: the author asserts that the field must move toward integration of these polarities if it is to abide within modern culture.

Haney, Theresa. *The Use of Dance/Movement Therapy with Adolescents in a Short-Term Inpatient Psychiatric Facility.* Hunter College, 1993.

Har-El Belach, Rivi. *The Psychological Implication of Moving in Different Planes.* Hunter College, 1991.

This study explores the relationship between three personality traits (risk-taking, self-esteem and social participation) and the use of different planes (sagittal, vertical and horizontal). An analysis was made of the results of three personality tests given to a group of dance therapy students.

Harmon, Nicole K. *Race, Culture, and Ethnicity, as it Relates to Dance Therapy from an African-American Perspective.* Hunter College, 1994.

The purpose of this study is to help bridge the gaps in the dance therapy modality when working with African-Americans. Through the examination of issues pertaining to the African-American culture, we see how the culture manifests in the therapy session when given space to present. Equally important to the therapeutic alliance is the dance therapist's own awareness of the issues that are provoked and manifested when working with African-Americans.

The study focuses on an analysis of the author's interactions with other African-American group members in a dance therapy session. A videotaped dance therapy session is analyzed using "Analysis of Interaction in Movement Sessions" (AIMS) which identifies behavioral and system elements to examine these interactions. By extracting and identifying these interactions, personal insight is gained by creating a welcoming environment in which African-American group members can interact and communicate. It is the conjecture of the author that an African-American dance therapist has greater interactions with those group members who are also African-American in a pluralistic group.

Hartstein, Jennifer Leigh. *Implementing Dance/Movement Therapy with an HIV+ Population: A Pilot Project.* Allegheny University of the Health Sciences, (formerly Hahnemann University, 1994.

The objective of this thesis is to propose that dance/movement therapy is an effective treatment modality when working with an HIV (human immunodeficiency virus) infected population. It suggests that dance/movement therapy can be equally as productive as verbal psychotherapy. The premise/assumption is that through the release of emotional responses within the movement sessions, an HIV+ individual will be more aware of his/her feelings, thus being able to deal with them more effectively. The author suggests that dance/movement therapy will have a positive effect on the negative emotions and physical states associated with being HIV positive. Two pilot dance/movement therapy sessions were conducted with clients who were infected and/or affected by the human immunodeficiency virus. The goals of these sessions were to reduce stress, release tension, increase energy levels (reducing fatigue), and to provide a safe, supportive environment in which to express emotions. A questionnaire was given asking participants for feedback on their movement experience. Comments were positive with regard to the stated goals. This population, especially in an inner city, has a great deal of life needs that outweigh psychotherapeutic needs. Suggestions as to how to develop a program are included.

Hayes, Jill S. *A Dance-Movement Therapy Study of a Young Girl with Relationship Difficulties.* Laban Centre for Movement and Dance, 1992.

Hayes, Laura. *The Use of Dance Movement Therapy With Dually Diagnosed Patients in a Short Term Psychiatric Facility.* Hunter College, 1994.

To support the use of dance/movement therapy with dually diagnosed patients in a short-term psychiatric facility, this paper reviews the symptoms and the treatment of dually diagnosed patients. It focuses on dance/movement therapy interventions to support the development and implementation of a dance/movement therapy group. A description of the dance/movement therapy group is presented along with the results of the group experience. A questionnaire is included which aided in monitoring patients' responses to the group. Interventions focus on developing healthy coping mechanisms, self-esteem and trust in dance/movement therapy groups to help patients re-enter society.

Hazama, Emi. *Case Study of Mentally Retarded Male in Dance/Movement Therapy.* Hunter College, 1992.

This is a study on the use of dance therapy in the treatment of John, a mentally retarded senior male. Individual dance therapy sessions helped this isolated patient participate in group dance therapy sessions and interact with others. The discussion focuses on the dance therapy goals for John in individual and group sessions. His sense of humor, motivation, abilities in communication and basic movement skills improved. Modification of his behaviors show him as trainable. Through the use of dance therapy, John's anger was expressed and his interactional skills improved.

Hedson, Alys Beth. *Dance/Movement Therapy and Behavior Therapy for the Autistic Child: A Literature Review.* Allegheny University of the Health Sciences (formerly Hahnemann University), 1995.

The literature review focuses on two therapeutic fields, dance/movement therapy and behavior therapy. It reviews their contributions as treatment modalities for the autistic child in support of a milieu treatment program. The review discusses similarities and contrasts among the two therapies. The following conclusions are made: the changes and modifications of the symptom descriptions of autism reflect the varying treatment approaches that are currently being practiced; the literature shows that the treatment of dance/movement therapy has increased the autistic child's capacity to relate to his/her environment; the child's repertoire of movement behaviors and emotions have expanded as a result of the combination of the therapeutic relationship and the kinesthetic process as reinforcement of the movement utilized in dance/movement therapy; and the treatment of behavior therapy has shown to increase the autistic child's academic (IQ) and self-help skills. Differences were found among the techniques used by the two therapies. An interface was found in the area of formulating goals. Both treatment modalities introduce and expand new skills with which the autistic child can better cope with his/her environment.

Henry, Jennifer T. *Object Relations and Dance/Movement Therapy.* Goucher College, 1993.

The purpose of this study is to explore the way in which an object relations theoretical approach to psychotherapy manifests itself in the theoretical and practical applications to dance/movement therapy with the adult psychiatric population. The areas of literature reviewed include: general theories in the development of the self, object relations theory and psychotherapy, dance/movement therapy theory and practice, and the integrated material on the treatment of psychiatric adults through object relations-based dance/movement therapy.

Ten dance/movement therapists who use an object relations approach to the treatment of adults were contacted. Eight were interviewed. Information on the therapist's facility and services, clinical and theoretical approach to assessment, individual therapy, group therapy, and goals, is provided.

There is a discussion of the data collected on object relations' clinical and theoretical applications to dance/movement therapy. The interviews revealed that while there exists a variety of possible movement characteristics in adults for any one developmental phase, there is a common quality reflective of the developmental task of that phase. Clinical interventions were based on developmental tasks specific to each phase of separation/individuation. The results of the study reflect the broad nature with which object relations must be interpreted through dance/movement therapy with the adult patient.

Future research can further support and expand the findings of this study by providing observable examples of the theoretical concepts.

Henson, Kathryn Beth Heidi. *The Utilization of Touch in the Psychotherapeutic Relationship Specific to Dance Movement Therapy.* Naropa Institute, 1992.

This thesis investigates the use of touch as a therapeutic intervention in dance/movement therapy. It is an inquiry into dance/movement therapists' training, current practices and beliefs. Along with awareness, this paper strives to clarify and define appropriate touch contact to the benefit of the dance/movement therapy profession; educationally, morally, ethically and legally. The literature review contains information on the skin; imprinting, learning and marasmus; healing nature and historical perspective; dominance, power, sex and abuse; therapeutic issues, ethical and legal concerns; and theorists and their theories. Local, in-person interviews were conducted followed by a nationwide questionnaire. These surveys explored process, procedure and therapeutic intent, concerns, suggestions for future training, and the impact of this inquiry. Ideas for future research, training, and the conclusions were extrapolated from the literature search, the survey, and the author's thoughts and experiences. The appendix includes a copy of the questionnaire, the American Dance Therapy Association Code of Ethics, and a checklist for evaluating personal morality and ethical style.

Hey, Jackie. *One-to One: A Journey of Discovery into the Experience of Dance Movement Therapy.* Laban Centre London, 1996.

This thesis began with an interest in finding out about the experience of one-to-one dance movement therapy for both the therapist and the client. Present scientific research methods were unsuitable for the type of enquiry the author wished to conduct. Therefore, before it was possible to go ahead with the discovery process, an alternative method of inquiry was needed. On reviewing the literature, it was found that dance movement therapists and other creative arts therapists are struggling with trying to be accepted by aiming to scientifically and empirically 'prove' the worth of their work by focussing on charts, scales and theories. But this 'clinification syndrome' has not worked due to the fact that the essence of dance movement therapy and other creative arts therapies are not within charts and theories but in experience, and the psychological change resulting from this experience.

This study documents the discovery and exploration of a more favourable method of enquiry. This method makes use of poetry, storytelling, drawing and diaries as a way of entering the experience of dance movement therapy. The author employs this method to further understand experiences within dance movement therapy and the resultant changes within both the client and herself as therapist. The results of this enquiry are presented in the form of chapters exploring the experience of progression of three themes. A further outcome of this work is that it enabled the writer to identify and begin to formulate an understanding of her personal way of working as a dance movement therapist. This is based on the belief that people have an intuitive healing process which has effect without the need for interpretation. This method of enquiry was not only a useful way of finding out about dance movement therapy process but it also became an integral part of the therapy process itself.

Higgins, Susan. *Integration of Movement/Expressive Arts: Case Study of a Suicidal Adolescent.* Antioch/New England Graduate School, 1993.

This thesis explores the use of individual movement/expressive arts therapy for the outpatient treatment of a suicidal adolescent. A case history of a 13 year old girl is presented describing the integration of movement/expressive arts therapy as the primary therapeutic intervention during 16 individual sessions over a four month period. Multimodal expressive arts therapy integrated with a psychoanalytic approach to movement therapy reduces the risk of suicide by offering active expression, containment and completion of emotions in a safe, non-judgmental environment, followed by the development of age-appropriate alternatives for coping with stress. Further research, study and publication are needed to explore and document the use of a movement/expressive arts therapy approach to individual short-term treatment for outpatient suicidal adolescents.

Hill, Heather. *An Attempt to Describe and Understand Moments of Experiential Meaning within the Dance Therapy Process for a Patient with Dementia.* Latrobe University (Australia), 1995. (UMI Dissertation Services).

This thesis reports an attempt to describe and understand moments of experiential meaning within the dance therapy process for a patient with dementia. It documents an attempt to develop a methodology which could adequately grasp the complexities of such an experience. A phenomenological approach with its emphasis on allowing the phenomenon to reveal itself through multiple perspectives seemed appropriate. However, while phenomenology influenced the format of the dance therapy sessions as well as the constitution and analysis of the data, ultimately a hermeneutic analysis was employed for further explication of the material. The study consisted of four individual dance therapy sessions with an 85 year old patient with moderate dementia. The researcher/therapist worked improvisationally and a music therapist provided improvised music. After the sessions, all of which were videotaped, the patient was videotaped viewing the dance session video, in order to obtain her verbal or nonverbal responses. The focus was on the "significant moments" selected intuitively as moments which seemed high points of the session. A naive description was made on which an adaptation of Giorgi's four phase method of analysis was applied. Certain foci, such as energy flow, were identified and individually described. In time, it became clear that the written descriptions alone were insufficient and that reflection would need to cover all the material from multiple sources and perspectives. The data was further explicated by reference to writings on dance therapy, dance aesthetics, and the philosophical concept of the embodied self, and Sack's neurological writings on the awakened self.

The conclusions were that the patient was not only transformed within the dance session and able to re-create aspects of her old self, but also underwent, through the experience as a whole (the dance and the reflection upon it facilitated by the video viewing), a change in awareness through which she reintegrated the past with the present and, in her words, came "out of the cupboard... into the brightness."

Hiller, Corinna A. *Dance Therapy at the Momentum AIDS Project: A Study of Expected Outcomes for an HIV+ Group.* Hunter College, 1996.

People with HIV can benefit from participating in dance therapy. Five dance therapy sessions were held at The Momentum AIDS Project with men in the symptomatic and asymptomatic stages of HIV infection. Nine standard expected dance therapy outcomes for an HIV+ group were created from the work of Comer (1992), Hartstein (1994), and Coburn (1995): 1) Express and accept all emotion 2) Self awareness 3) Reassess identity 4) Explore self-esteem 5) Explore conflict and psychic growth 6) Social support 7) Explore developmental needs 8) Develop trust 9) Learn coping mechanisms and how to meet needs.

Analysis of videotapes and group leader's logs from the sessions found that all nine outcomes were experienced in a least two sessions and six outcomes were experienced in every session. Participants' responses to questionnaires, administered after the five sessions, identified eight out of the nine outcomes, excluding only exploring conflict and psychic growth.

Himmelgreen, Carolyn. *Dream, Dance and Myth.* Hunter College, 1992.

This paper shows how dreams can be brought to conscious awareness through movement and myth. The literature review includes different theories and methods of dreamwork. Sigmund Freud discovered that dreams belonged to the unconscious. He viewed dreams as an expression of wish fulfillment and repressed sexuality. Carl Jung provided a more universal way of perceiving the world by introducing the "collective unconscious" wherein existed the world of archetypes, symbols, and personality types. Jung's theory of archetypal psychology is further expanded on by theorists using a feminist perspective and process work, who draw on the relationship between body symptoms and dreams. Dance therapists integrated Jung's "active imagination" into dance therapy as a way of facilitating the process of individuation. Psycho-dramatists used psychodrama to reenact real life situations as an active form of therapy to release emotions and create a catharsis. Dreamwork methods are used by theorists working with groups and individuals as a way of working with dreams without a professional facilitator.

The author established a dream group, combining theories and methods in order to find out what does or does not work when "moving the dream." The techniques are borrowed from Ullman, Faraday, Moreno, and Perls but the perspective is predominantly Jungian. The purpose of this case study was to find out how the enactment of dreams can lead to further self-awareness.

The methodology includes a total of five dream enactments. The group consisted of three second-year students from the graduate dance/movement therapy program at Hunter College. One participant is the dreamer (myself) the other two are participants in the enactments. We met on five occasions and each session lasted from one to two hours. Moving the dream helped to increase my insight. Recreating the dream images enabled me to connect my inner life to my outer existence. The dream images, gestures, and posturing stirred up feelings that might have stayed dormant. Myth used in conjunction with interpreting the dream enactments helped to validate my experiences and bring them to a more universal level of understanding.

Hollander, Margot E. *When the Therapist is Female: Role Conflict and Counter-Transference with a Male Patient During Group Dance Therapy Sessions.* Hunter College, 1991.

This is a case study of a female therapist's counter-transferential reactions to a male patient during group dance therapy sessions. The study seeks to identify the relationship between the patient's behaviors and the therapist's reactions, explore the possible origins of the therapist's counter-transference, and to highlight the ways in which the tensions between the roles of the therapist and female may have contributed to her on-going and pressured reactions.

The literature review presents a survey of differing viewpoints about countertransference with particular emphasis on the meanings, clinical significance and uses that individual theorists attribute to this term. It explores the relationship between gender and countertransference by examining and contrasting the roles of the women in contemporary western society and in psychotherapeutic treatment approaches. Areas of role conflict and subsequent countertransference are identified. In addition, the literature review highlights the immediacy of counter-transferential reactions in dance therapy and surveys the literature within the field.

The therapist's counter-transferential reactions were culled from process notes from ten dance therapy sessions using indicators agreed upon in the literature. These reactions fell into four categories: cognitive, emotional, behavioral, and motoric responses. The reactions were then examined for attitudes and behaviors reflective of role conflict and organized into further four categories: nurturance, personal authority, sexuality, and aggression. The discussion of the case material focuses on the ways in which the therapist was and was not able to resolve her counter-transference in these thematic areas, and concludes that her counter-transferential responses stemmed from conflicts between her professional role and her internalized feminine role prescriptions.

Howard, Katherine. *Grounding Luis: Individual Dance Therapy with a Patient Diagnosed as Schizophrenic.* Hunter College, 1995.

This is a case study of an individual diagnosed with chronic schizophrenia. It traces seven dance therapy sessions in which the author utilizes a movement ritual designed to help ground the patient in reality. Specifically, it looked for a relationship between physical grounding and an increase in reality-based verbalizations. The movement sequence chosen incorporated early developmental movement patterns and Lab analysis concepts of weight and space effort as interpreted by Bartenieff. Results indicate that such a structure may be a useful tool in helping to heal the body/mind split characteristic of schizophrenia.

Hrushovski, Tammy. *The Individuation Process of MBD Children Through Dance/Movement Therapy.* Lesley College Graduate School, 1993.

This study is about the individuation process through dance therapy of children with minimal brain dysfunction. The development of motor abilities and movement expression is strongly connected to the development of sense of self. This can be clearly seen when working with MBD children. The deficiencies in their motor functioning influence their psychic development from birth on, and their emotional disturbances in turn influence their motor ability.

The MBD child can reexperience his/her object-relations development through movement expressed in the relationship that evolves between him/her and the dance therapist. Within their relationship, the practicing of the patient's motor skills and his/her independence is an important aspect of the child's development towards acquiring a sense of a separate and coherent self. A case study of group therapy with two six year old girls who suffer from minimal brain dysfunction is presented to illustrate a way of working with these children. Theories of MBD disorder, object relations and dance therapy are elaborated to provide the theoretical background for this work.

Huber, Wendy Ferris. *Marian Chace: Her Work and the Perceptions of Those Who Knew Her.* Goucher College, 1991.

The purpose of this project is to examine the work of dance/movement therapy innovator Marian Chace specifically addressing the questions: what were the assumptions, principles, goals and process of dance therapy pioneer Marian Chace according to her own writings; and how did others perceive Chace as a therapist and as Chace the person. Elements of Marian Chace's personal and professional life are examined using her own writings, and the impressions and experiences of those who knew, studied, and worked with Ms. Chace.

A videotape was constructed consisting of a demonstration group illustrating her work. It includes parts of interviews with two of Chace's former students. Five other former students of Chace were interviewed and the commonalities and differences among them analyzed, seeking to understand what made Chace an effective therapist. The author found this project to be about commitment. Commitment to the patients and to dance as a healing profession appeared to be the key element that contributed to Chace's powerful presence.

Hudak, Karen M. *Gender in Affective Experiences and Expressions in Dance/Movement Therapy.* Goucher College, 1992.

The purpose of this study is to discover if there are any similarities or differences between men and women in terms of their affective experiences and expressions in dance/movement therapy. Literature in the areas of the development of men and women, affect, and dance/movement therapy are reviewed. The methodology involved eight weekly dance/movement therapy sessions with three men and five women which were led by a registered dance/movement therapist. Criteria for the recruitment of subjects consisted of the following: no previous psychiatric hospitalization or psychiatric diagnoses, between the ages of 25 and 65 years old, born in the United States, no serious physical handicaps, and not currently involved in any type of therapy. At the end of each session, time was allotted for the subjects and the therapist to write in journals. The journal entries were responses to specific guidelines regarding the subjects' affective experiences during each session.

The guidelines asked about specific emotions that the subjects may or may not have experienced, such as anger, sadness, fear, joy, defending against emotions, anxiety, excitement, and others. The therapist noted observations of the subjects' demonstrations of emotions in each session, and noted with which gender these occurred. The results showed that there were both similarities and differences in the experiences and expressions of affect for men and women. The females reported more experiences of emotion, with a wider range of affect than the males. The males and females expressed many similar emotions, but the therapist perceived the genders as expressing distinct feelings too, such as sarcasm in the males and dependency in the females. The literature supports that males tend to be less aware of their emotional experiences than females and less likely to discuss these experiences. This is utilized as explanations for the results of this study.

Hudson, Kathleen A. *An Exploratory Study of the Use of Cotherapy in Dance/Movement Therapy.* Allegheny University of the Health Sciences (formerly Hahnernann University), 1992.

Cotherapy is a modality that is commonly used in the practice and training of dance/movement therapists. Although it is widely used there is little literature on the combination of these two modalities. Through the use of a questionnaire, this author conducted an exploratory, descriptive study on the general use of co-leading in the dance/ movement therapy modality and the opinions of the dance/movement therapists on this usage. The study sought a relationship between the extent of formal dance or movement training and reported perceived success of the movement cotherapy relationship. No significant relationship was found. Two other hypotheses were tested. One stated that those who were trained by coleading will report a perceived higher success rate in coleading than those who were not, and this hypothesis approached significance. The other stated the perceived success rates of the cotherapy relationship reported in dance/movement therapy groups will be higher than reported perceived success rates in general cotherapy relationships. This hypothesis proved highly significant.

Hugill, Tannis. *Somatic Approaches to the Treatment of Bulimia From the Perspective of a Wounded Healer.* Antioch/New England Graduate School, 1992.

In this thesis the author describes the use of somatic interventions in the treatment of a client with bulimia nervosa over a twelve week period. A synthesis of bioenergetic exercises, dance therapy, and drama therapy was utilized. Because of the limited time and experimental nature of this project, the author worked under supervision as well as in association with the client's primary therapist. Presented is the author's own history of involvement with and recovery from an eating disorder and a brief history of the etiology of anorexia and bulimia nervosa. Interviews with five therapists using similar approaches support the value of these somatic treatment strategies. The twelve sessions conducted are described and summarized. The client experienced significant positive bodily responses, and reported increased understanding of her relationship to bulimia. Given the short time frame of our work, the outcome of this study supports the hypothesis that somatic approaches to treatment can be beneficial.

Hurst, Stacey M. *Dance/Movement Therapy Case Study Analysis Using the Relational Model and Kestenberg Movement Profile.* Columbia College, 1996.

This thesis retrospectively analyzes the relational development of an adolescent who was involved in one-to-one dance/movement therapy session over a six month period. It shows how the use of individual long term dance/movement therapy, and more specifically the empathic movement relationship between patient and therapist supported this adolescent's development from a two dimensional non-relating body posture/psyche to a three dimensional posture of relating. The analysis bridges three models: 1) Dance/movement therapy (D/MT), 2) the Relational model (RM) and 3) the Kestenberg Movement Profile (KMP). It shows how the use of these models in combination supported the client's establishment of trust between himself and the author, awareness of his emotions and verbalization of same to others, and an increase in self-esteem and self-image. Additionally, the Relational Model allowed this writer to recognize the unconscious process of connection and disconnection due to transference and countertransference on a body awareness level. The purpose of this paper is to illuminate the power of the therapeutic movement relationship, created on a body felt level, between the therapist and patient. This case study serves as an example of how this process occurs as well as providing an example of an approach to building a therapeutic relationship in a one-to-one dance/movement therapy session.

Hyle, Danielle. *Stress Management and Body Awareness Exercises Implemented into Exercise Regimen of Phase II Cardiac Rehabilitation Patients: An Experimental Case Study.* Lesley College Graduate School, 1996.

The recent literature about cardiac outpatient rehabilitation clearly shows that both stress management classes and exercise programs help patients recover from cardiac trauma. It has become evident that these components function independently of one another with no focus on integrated healing. One program deals with the physiological recovery while the other deals with the psycho-social aspect of the patient. It is the purpose of this thesis to examine the use of dance-movement therapy techniques of stress management and body awareness exercises within the physical conditioning workouts of Phase II of Cardiac Rehabilitation. It is believed that by using Bartenieff Fundamentals (1980) exercises during the physical conditioning workouts, a greater consistency in heart rate and blood pressure would occur in the subject of this single case study. The results show the Fundamentals (Bartenieff. 1980) exercises supported the success of this patient. It is also theorized that a larger sense of body-mind integration occurred during his cycle of Phase II of Cardiac Rehabilitation.

Irving, Deborah. *Depression and Dance Therapy*. Hunter College, 1976.
The paper concerns itself with the etiology, symptoms and treatment of depression in older persons. It statistically validates the hypothesis that time structured dance therapy with moderately depressed senior citizens will significantly reduce their degree of depression.

Isecke, Martina. *Dance Movement Group Therapy with Rheumatoid Arthritis Patients in View of Psychosomatic Concepts of Organic and Chronic Illness*. Laban Centre for Movement and Dance, 1995.

Isis, Kali Bird. *Who Will Hold The Broken Hearted? A Guide To Working With Parents Whose Babies Have Died*. Antioch/New England Graduate School, 1991.
This thesis presents an examination of the grieving process in parents whose baby has died at, during, or just prior to birth. It is argued that Western culture resists supporting the parents as they grieve and offers little support in allowing resolution to occur. The expressive arts therapist is presented as a possible shaman or guide to the grieving parents. Techniques such as active imagination and ritual are considered as means of travelling within the unconscious where the archetypal grief may be encountered and healed. A brief examination of shamanism is considered and compared to the traditional psychotherapy offered to most grieving parents in Western society. Especially considered is the bereaved mother's process through her grief and lack of support. Suggestions for the expressive arts therapist working with grieving parents are presented and the art work and poetry of a number of surviving parents is represented. The author's own experience as a grieving mother and her use of the expressive arts in her healing is considered. It is argued that by fully surrendering to the process of grieving and allowing the wounds to be healed, the griever and the expressive arts therapist who serves as guide can transform great pain into a greater universal peace.

Jackson, Sarah. *Young People Who Have Emotional and Severe Learning Difficulties—The Case for Dance Movement Therapy*. Laban Centre for Movement and Dance, 1993.

Jacoby, Rita. *Toward an Integrated Theory of Dance/Movement Therapy*. Antioch/New England Graduate School, 1993.
This thesis examines the theoretical developments in dance/movement therapy and proposes a framework for an integrated theory. In the course of its history, dance/movement therapy has developed a range of theoretical orientations, largely on the basis of psychological theories. Although this constitutes an important advance for the field, it has also led to a certain fragmentation as these theoretical developments have failed to attend to the special nature of the dance medium to systematically build the foundation of dance/movement therapy. The theoretical model set forth in this thesis bases its assumptions on the properties of dance and its interface with individual psychology. It looks at the psychology of dance/movement in terms of the dynamic relationship between experience and its symbolized expression, the interplay of which is seen as the root of the transformative process

in dance/movement therapy. This model is then used to organize dance/movement therapy techniques according to their functions within the therapeutic process. Finally, the spectrum of intervention techniques is applied to the differential treatment of psychopathologies, integrating various theoretical approaches within a developmental framework.

Janco, Orit. *Healing in Water: Dance/Movement Therapy in Water With The Chronic Pain Population.* Antioch/New England Graduate School, 1991.

The primary purpose of this thesis is to explore the benefits and treatment of dance/movement therapy (DMT) with the chronic pain population in a swimming pool setting. Due to a lack of published literature on this subject, most of the data in this descriptive research paper has been compiled from personal experiences, correspondence and interviews with dance/movement therapists working in the water medium in addition to a patient questionnaire. Patients' responses affirm their participation in these groups. Patients describe the benefits in terms of reducing their pain, anxiety and body tensions, as well as increasing their mood, range of movement and social skills. Conclusions are formulated based on observations of these DMT groups in water and on patients' experiences. Recommendations for further applications and studies, empirical or other are determined.

Jasperse, Kristin. *The Movement Dynamics of Shame: Exploring Shame as an Addictive Process.* Naropa Institute, 1990.

The literature review includes definitions, descriptions including the physiological, and treatment approaches toward shame. In researching the topic of shame, the author was intrigued by the description of the characteristic downward spiral associated with the felt experience of shame. The downward spiral of shame occurs when the individual experiences an intense moment of felt exposure. The person has the distinct sensation of being pulled downward. As this happens, the individual is immersed further and further into their shame to the point of being totally engulfed within the shame experience. One client often talked of feeling caught in such a "downward spiral". This client's description,coupled with the literature's explanation of the spiral and her own personal experience point to the possibility of shame being an addictive process whose purpose is to distance the person from awareness of their direct experience. Thus, identifying the bodily manifestations of shame and introducing the experience and function of shame as an addictive process in movement is the focus of this thesis.

Jingu, Kyoko. *Cross-Cultural Issues in Dance Therapy for Japanese Clients.* Hunter College, 1996.

The basic assumption is that cultural values effect the way people respond to dance therapy sessions. By reviewing the literature, the Japanese and mental health, Japanese psychological constructs and its relation to interpersonal expressive behavior, and Japanese ways of understanding body, movement and dance, the author attempts to elucidate effective use of dance therapy and particular considerations when working with Japanese clients.

Johns, Stephanie Denise. *African Dance Ritual Elements And Their Clinical Applications In Dance/Movement Therapy.* Goucher College, 1993.

The purpose of this study is to examine the benefits that African dance ritual elements may have for dance/movement therapy in terms of providing additional means toward therapeutic interventions as well as a conceptual framework for further interpretations of the dance/movement therapy process. The literature review includes the history, goals, principles, and elements of dance/movement therapy. African dance rituals are discussed based on their history, function, and prominent elements.

The information from this is combined into an integrative chapter uncovering the similarities and differences between dance/movement therapy and African dance rituals. The elements found to be common between both disciplines (structure, rhythm, symbolism, and imagery) are recreated based on their function within African dance rituals and hypothetically incorporated into dance/movement therapy sessions. Detailed descriptions of each element and its clinical application to various age groups and clinical populations are presented.

The fact that these clinical examples are hypothetical makes it hard to state generalizations about the findings. However, it does appear that the elements of structure, rhythm, imagery, and symbolism in African dance rituals are beneficial for dance/movement therapy, and can be incorporated into the dance/movement therapy process. The ritual elements of imagery and symbolism seemed to provide additional interventions and interpretations that were different from what already exists in dance/movement therapy.

Kahlen, Melanie Renate. *"Stuckness" in the Psychotherapeutic Process: The Confrontation with the Unknown.* Naropa Institute, 1995.

This thesis investigates the phenomenon and dynamics of "stuckness" in the psychotherapeutic process. Varied psychological theories concerning the causes and handling of client stuckness are drawn together in the review of literature. A survey is performed to assess attitudes on psychological stuckness held by dance/movement therapists. Six local, in-person interviews were conducted with dance therapists, psychotherapists, and movement teachers as the basis for a subsequent questionnaire. The nationwide questionnaire responded to by twenty-one dance/movement therapists was designed to identify therapists' theoretical approaches and judgements on the causes and appearances of stuckness in the clients as well as in themselves and techniques they prefer in dealing with either client and/or therapist stuckness.

Results indicate that stuckness can be considered a useful stage in the process of change. It functions as a regulator to protect a person in different ways in the face of conflicting experiences which are perceived as threatening. The predominant emotional, cognitive, and perceptual causes of stuckness are discussed. Essential goals as well as numerous approaches, techniques, and interventions to work with and through client and therapist stuckness are reviewed. The potentially negative connotation and impact of the term "stuckness" is addressed.

Karash, A. *Jimmy and Peggy: Analysis of Two Dance Therapy Sessions with Autistic Children.* Hunter College, 1977.

Kasovac, Nicholas. *Possible Etiologies for Disorders in which Patients Exhibit Body Boundary Difficulties.* University of California, Los Angeles, 1993. (SP)

Kaspi, Osnat. *Moving Through Creative Blocks: Facilitating The Creative Process With DMT.* Antioch/New England Graduate School, 1993.

This work is a journey through the stages and blocks of the creative process. The focus of this work is facilitating the creative process with dance/movement therapy (DMT) and moving through creative blocks. The basic philosophical view points are that life is a creative process and that in the essence of our being is the ability to be creative. Therapy is also a creative process of finding ways to cope with problems and challenges and to generate new insights and ideas for living a continuous and flowing life-journey. Life's problems and likewise a client's presenting dilemmas, are viewed as creative blocks to living and to development.

Movement and sensation are essential in creativity and in the resolution of creative blocks.

Awareness (metacreativity), fear of the unknown and tension between polarities are explored as necessary and basic elements in understanding and overcoming creative blocks. The literature on the topics of creativity, the creative process and the various creative blocks is reviewed. Various experiential DMT techniques to enhance self-awareness, facilitate expression of imagination, overcome the fear of the unknown and the tension between polarities, such as improvisation and creative visualization, are suggested in order to resolve creative blocks. The inherent value of blocks is also examined.

Keck, Anneka Emily. *The Cry of the Soul in Flesh: An Alternative View and Treatment of First Break Psychosis.* Naropa Institute, 1996.

Not all of the psychic states diagnosed by our culture as mental illness are either pathological or abnormal but can be likened to a physical illness with both a functionality and a probable cure. The fundamental allowance of pathology as a temporary state of an organism in healing flux derives from the paradigm of naturopathic vs. alllopathic medicine. A holistic view of mental illness allows for a holistic cure.

Insanity is a natural stage in the evolution of the mind, perhaps not a necessary stage, but nevertheless insanity itself is neither abnormal, chronic, or inalterable. So often the diagnosis of mental illness is given as an absolute- like the diagnosis of a terminal illness such as metastasized cancer whose symptoms can be controlled but whose cause is now inexorably mapped into the body and cannot be treated or cured. This thesis proposes the hypothesis that mental illness as a permanent diagnosis of a largely incurable state is a complete and total fallacy.

Kennedy, James Ryan. *Alchemical Hypnotherapy and Hypnotherapeutic Techniques in Dance/Movement Therapy.* Naropa Institute, 1993.

This theoretical examination explores how the application of hypno-therapeutic techniques and the specific process of alchemical hypnotherapy can be used to accentuate the therapeutic interventions of dance/movement therapy. Through the blending of these two therapeutic modalities, an increased awareness of subconscious processing and expression is anticipated, allowing for a broader perspective on a client's presenting issues and a clearer understanding of the possible directions for treatment.

Alchemical hypnotherapy uses an interactive trance state to access people, events, and parts of the self within the subconscious mind, providing insight into personal healing and transformation. The psychotherapeutic process of dance/movement therapy is the avenue by which embodiment, expression, and integration of direct experience occurs through movement. Both of these psychotherapeutic approaches employ the imaginative processes of precognitive, right-brain thinking and encourage the immediate and direct experiencing of emotions and sensations in the body.

The premise of this work is that the integration of these two processes allows for a greater degree of therapeutic change. The connection is based on the supposition that an understanding of alchemical hypnotherapy provides the dance/movement therapist an increased knowledge and facility with accessing, identifying, and employing altered states of consciousness in the therapeutic process. Through the combination of theoretical research, clinical studies, and personal experience, a positive relationship is shown demonstrating that the alchemical processes can be applied in a dance/movement therapy session to inform, guide, and enhance the psychotherapeutic process.

Keyeski, Julie. *Moving Beyond Therapy: Expanding the Container of Dance/Movement.* California State University, Hayward, 1996.

The author encourages the profession of dance/movement therapy to expand its focus to include wellness and prevention. Literature reveals that therapy is limited in its ability to attend to mental health and programs which stress wellness and prevention are thought to be more efficacious. "Dance for Wellness" is presented as an extension of dance/movement therapy that could be utilized in schools, community programs, and employee health programs.

Khodl, Nada Anna. *The Goddess Within Dance/Movement Therapy.* Goucher College, 1993.

The purpose of this study is to explore the possibilities for the use of goddess imagery in dance/movement therapy as catalysts for women to gain greater self-esteem. The author investigates how these two are used together to stimulate a growth process that leads to associations of personal material with goddess images. Literature in the areas of women and self-esteem, myth, and dance/movement therapy are reviewed. The literature on women and self-esteem comprises the areas of women through the ages and the psychology of women today. The literature on myth comprises its definitions, importance and functions of the myth today, mythology and psychology, the goddess, and current interest in the goddess. The dance/movement therapy section comprises an introduction, definition, and a discussion of its history, principles, goals, and process with a focus on those aspects which relate to the topic.

A dance/movement therapy group was conducted by this researcher. Ten women were recruited based on these criteria: a) between the ages of 21 and 65; b) no previous or current history of psychiatric illnesses or hospitalizations; c) in need of improved self-esteem as evidenced by the Index of Self-Esteem (ISE) (Hudson, 1991); d) a commitment to attending all eight sessions; and e) no serious physical illnesses or disabilities. Seven sessions were run by the author, five of which incorporated the goddess myths. The first session was used as an orientation to the study and the final session was used as a closing group. Results were assessed through the use of subjective measures. Journals were kept by both the author and the subjects according to specific guidelines.

The results are reported in three ways: a) through the perspective of the author; b) through the perspective of the subjects and; c) through charts which highlight subject results. The results show that at least seven out of ten subjects improved their self-esteem in varying ways and to varying degrees. The author interprets these results for individual subjects, discussing the most notable changes that occurred in the sessions. One interpretation is that the subjects were able to discover the means within themselves to continue building their self-esteem.

Kinni, Eleftheria. *A Review of the Problems Encountered in the Study and Management of Depression and the Implications for Dance Movement Therapy.* Laban Centre for Movement and Dance, 1992.

Kinsey, Victoria. *Applications of Dance Therapy for Adult Survivors of Childhood Sexual Abuse.* Hunter College, 1994.

This paper examines the applications of dance therapy theory and practice for the population of adult survivors of sexual abuse. The author reviews literature related specifically to sexual abuse including studies of prevalent theories about associated risk factors, theories about perpetrators of sexual abuse and studies of its long term effects. A selection of treatment goals and methods are reviewed. Group therapy theory is presented, focusing on those aspects most relevant to the population. The author cites specific dance therapy studies and theoretical works concerned with related subjects. The author concludes that dance therapy has the potential to be an important part of the treatment of adult survivors of childhood sexual abuse. A number of recommendations concerning the use of dance therapy with this population are presented, along with suggestions for areas of future research of the subject.

Kitt, Alyce Lynn. *Anxiety-It's Effect on Client-Therapist Interaction.* Hunter College, 1983.

A dance therapy session in a day treatment center in Suffolk County was videotaped in order to analyze a therapist's responses as a group leader. Observation of the tape revealed distinct anxiety on the part of the therapist. A review of the literature includes definitions and origins of anxiety, physiological components and types of anxiety, and main theories of anxiety. Seven clients, three females and four males, of varied diagnoses participated in the videotaped session. Ten parameters were chosen to describe the interaction between client and therapist. Therapist anxiety occurred throughout the session and was evident through much touch, little use of eye contact, a preponderance of proximity, movement changes, and much directive verbalizations. The therapist used much control during this session to help relieve her level of anxiety. Therefore, the clients were allowed little initiation or independent behavior. The manner in which therapists react to undue stress, tension, and anxiety will have a major effect on the successful outcome of a dance therapy session.

Klotzkin, Jeannine L. *An Experiment Using Breath With Psychiatric Patients.* Hunter College, 1992.

This study examines the effect of breathing exercises and deep breathing on an in-patient psychiatric dance therapy session. The hypothesis is that patients who participate in breathing exercises will have deeper breathing and in a dance therapy session, the patients will be more energetic, more expressive, creative, interactive and have improved concentration. Patient's breathing was measured using a volumetric incentive spirometer, and it was recorded for three consecutive dance therapy sessions, before and after the session. Prior to the third session, the patients participated in 15 minutes of breathing exercises. The latter two sessions were videotaped and reviewed by raters. The results indicate that only two of the five patients had deeper breathing after the breathing exercises. One of the two patients achieved the hypothesized results, while the other actually achieved opposite results. Despite the fact that most patient's breathing did not change significantly, the group as a whole was more energetic, expressive, interactive, and better focused. Therefore, breathing exercises can be effective for deepening some patient's breathing, and they do have an effect on a dance therapy session.

Kohl, Mieke. *Listening to the Non-Verbal Self: The Experience of Those Combining Authentic Movement with Verbal Psychotherapy.* Smith College School for Social Work, 1996.

This research study was conducted to explore the benefits of combining Authentic Movement, a gentle body-oriented discipline, with traditional verbal psychotherapy. It was hypothesized that this movement work offers elements which verbal therapy lacks and could therefore enhance the therapy. It was also hypothesized that therapy could be a useful adjunct to those involved in Authentic Movement who wanted more than the discipline could offer.

In this qualitative, exploratory study, seven subjects, practiced in both disciplines were interviewed using a semi-structured interview guide. Participants were asked to describe their experiences with Authentic Movement and with verbal psychotherapy including the similarities and differences between the two therapeutic forms.

The findings reveal that for all seven subjects, Authentic Movement offered access not only to repressed bodily and pre-verbal memories, but also to other unconscious material not easily accessible through verbal means. New ways of moving often led to the discovery of previously untapped sources of health, strength and wholeness. Attending to the body's messages with an attitude of complete acceptance was found to be particularly beneficial to the physical and sexual abuse survivors in this study; they gradually came to feel more connected to and comfortable with their own bodies. For one survivor who gained virtually no benefits from verbal therapy, Authentic Movement provided a means to deep and lasting emotional and physical transformation. It was concluded that this body oriented practice can be an important adjunct to traditional therapy as well as a valuable modality itself.

Koshland, Lynn Marie. *Walks of Life: Dance/Movement Therapy and Socialization With the Isolated Elderly.* Goucher College, 1993.

The purpose of this project is to portray, verbally and visually, how dance/movement therapy decreases social isolation of the elderly. The literature reviews aging and the elderly, and literature of dance/movement therapy is discussed including an integration of dance/movement therapy as applied to the isolated elderly. An accompanying video serves as a visual representation of the integration. A description is given of the methodology of running the dance/movement therapy group and and the group's process as well as selecting video images for the final product and a narrative of the video.

The video "Walks of Life: Dance/Movement Therapy and Socialization with the Elderly," incorporates both educational and kinesthetic material. The intent of this video is to portray the principles, goals, and techniques used in dance/movement therapy in relation to socialization of the isolated elderly. A theme of continuity reflects the process of life review in dance/movement therapy. Images were selected from six dance/movement therapy sessions with a group of six older Americans in combination with gathered nature shots, music, and voice over. This combination creates an overall feeling tone of being old and demonstrates how dance/movement therapy can help the elderly to reclaim intimacy and socialization in their lives.

Kram, C. Debra. *"Will you come back & visit?" A Look at the Process of Termination for Ralik, A Latency Age Boy in Residential Care.* Hunter College, 1991.

After an extensive discussion of the literature on the latency age child, childhood depression, and issues related to the ending phase of therapy, this paper follows the termination process of one child, a latency age boy with depressive features as he struggles with the feelings evoked when his therapist, a social work/dance therapy intern, nears the ending phase of her internship.

Kwon, Eun Hee. *Foot Fetish Child and Dance/Movement Therapy: Vigorous Patterns of Movement and Part-object Concept and their Significant Implications in Developing Body-self Image and Object Relationship.* New York University, 1991.

An exploration of the significance of a vigorous movement pattern in a three years and nine month old child in relation to foot fetish, developing body self image and object relationship. The study was developed based on the psychoanalytic developmental frames of reference of Freud, Mahler, Winnicott, Greenacre, and Galenson and Rophe. A phenomenological method was used to present and analyze the data gathered over a fourteen month period of twice weekly individual movement therapy sessions. The study concludes that the fourteen month period of direct contact and intervention resulted in a decline of frequency of the child's fetishistic behaviors and improvement of body image and object relatedness.

Landau, Atara. *The Totent Tanze: A Death Dance as a Wedding Rite.* Hunter College, 1993.

This thesis examines the history and healing effects of a Jewish Chassidic wedding and festival dance. Parallels are drawn between dance therapy and the Death Dance, or as it is also called, "The Resurrection of the Dead Dance". The Death Dance serves as a catharsis for the bride and groom, the dancers and the community as a whole. The theory behind this thesis is that this dance would not have prevailed over centuries if it did not serve a basic emotional need. The dance supplied a metaphor representing ambivalence and fear during times of change and upheaval.

Larsen, Kris Eric. *The Coming Out Process and the Utilization of Dance/Movement Therapy as a Gay-Affirming Psychotherapy.* Naropa Institute, 1994.

This thesis is about homosexuality. It is an exploration of the experience of the gay male in a society where he is often looked upon with anger and denial. The author seeks to understand how he, as a gay therapist, can better facilitate the gay experience. In response to societal pressures many men in the gay community develop maladaptive self-hating behavior. He seeks how to assist the gay male, through dance/movement therapy and the utilization of the Healing Cycle, in shifting from the internalized homophobic question "Why am I gay?" to a self-actualized "I am gay." The process of socialization, identity formation and social bias is discussed in order to define a path for positive sexual development for gay males. Case studies illustrate how the techniques of the Healing Cycle can be utilized as a gay-affirming therapy.

Leahy, Dana. *The Dancer Inside the Therapist: Redefining Product vs. Process.* Columbia College Chicago, 1995.

This thesis is based on original research, bibliographic material, direct observation and personal interviews. The populations focused on were young adults in a therapeutic setting and children of various ages in a classroom setting.

There is an attempt to examine the similarities and differences between dance education and dance movement therapy. Having experienced and studies both approaches to dance, it has become clear that a dichotomy exists between movement as a therapeutic method and movement as a technique taught in dance class.

The following ideas are explored: 1) the history of dance, 2) the transition to dance therapy, 3) the structure of a "class", 4) the structure of a "group", 5) interviews regarding dance class and dance movement therapy group, 6) the similarities and differences between the two studies, and 7) process vs. product, the reasons and benefits of dance as therapy and dance as education.

The thesis not only chronicles the similarities and differences but how important it is to understand the roots and process of dance as history. To be a dance therapist, especially one who has been a teacher, it is important to come to terms with and appreciate the means by which dance movement therapy was born.

Lebeaux, Cathy Geier. *Outreach and Collaborative Relationship Building as Approaches To Bring Expressive Arts Therapists Into Schools And Communities: A Community Mental Health Center's Example.* Antioch/New England Graduate School, 1996.

Dance/movement and other expressive arts therapies are being underutilized by schools and communities. However at CMHC (a pseudonym for a community mental health agency), dance/movement and expressive arts therapies have expanded and become an important part of their counseling, assessment, and other mental health services. CMHC has an internal environment where expressive arts, the agency's need for more income and increased outreach and exposure in the community are all simultaneously supported and valued through collaborative working relationships. How communities, schools and other organizations are brought into this process is explored through interviews with school counselors and other professionals involved in these collaborative relationships with CMHC. It is proposed that this approach can be co-constructed in other agencies, adding much to the expansion and image of dance/movement and other expressive arts therapies, as well as creating more career opportunities.

Leeds, Mimi. *Breakdancing: A Cultural Phenomenon.* Hunter College, 1985.

This paper presents an historical perspective on dance as a cultural and personal statement as derived from the existing literature. Dance is examined through five different categories. The five categories are: dance as ritual, dance as recreation, dance as education for the group experience, dance as a means for emotional release and dance as a vehicle for personal reflection for the individual experience.

Breakdancing, a contemporary form of street dance, is described through personal observation, and through the perspectives of breakdancers, inner-city adolescents and several authors who have explored the breakdancing phenomenon. The meaning of breakdancing is derived through examining the relationship of breakdancing to the above-mentioned general categories of dance expression. Through this evaluation, the impact of the breakdancing statement is acknowledged. A video tape is included in this project which illustrates the process and meaning generated through a workshop on breakdancing.

This paper explores the implications of breakdancing as a vehicle for therapeutic intervention. Here, my role as a dance therapist is described, highlighting the use of dance therapy training to generate non-traditional group format. The therapeutic process is explored, creating a model to work with cultural groups and age ranges which are dramatically different from the therapists personal background.

Leighton, Felicia E. *Creative Selves-In-Relation In Taoist Tai Chi And Dance/Movement Therapy.* Antioch/New England Graduate School, 1993.

Literature pertaining to community building, the self-in-relation and Taoist Tai Chi is employed for a theoretical synthesis with applications to dance/movement therapy. The social oppression of body-felt experience and creativity is associated with the decay of community and relational ability. Dance/movement therapy is supported as a means of rekindling this kind of expression. Movement is discussed as an imperative component of relational communication which can foster the formation of community. Taoist Tai Chi is examined for its spiritual principles that support relationship and community, as well as its physical means of restoring range to the capacity for relational movement. A relationship between creativity and connectedness is suggested in this synthesis of dance/movement therapy, community building and Taoist Tai Chi, three theories that support development of the self-in-relation as a means to individual and social health.

LeMessurier, Claire. *Child Sexual Abuse and Dance/Movement Therapy: A Case Study.* Antioch/New England Graduate School, 1990.

Evidence of child sexual abuse is becoming increasingly prevalent. An overview of recent literature on the subject examines the effects of child sexual abuse and treatment strategies in verbal and movement therapies. A case study of a latency age female survivor of sexual abuse is described. There is a detailed summary of individual dance therapy sessions over a period of fifteen months and a description of a twelve week long movement therapy group in which the client participated. The process of therapy is discussed and evaluated. An argument is made for the use of dance/movement therapy as a primary mode of treatment for child survivors of sexual abuse.

Lemon, Janet. *The Use of Dance/Movement Therapy in Professional Sport: A Kestenberg Movement Profile of Joe Montana.* Antioch/New England Graduate School, 1990.

This is a case study of one professional athlete, using the Kestenberg Movement Profile, an observational and analytic tool utilized in the field of dance/movement therapy. Videotaped football games, one commercial and one post-game interview were viewed to collect data of one quarterback's (Joe Montana) movement. In this paper the results are analyzed and compared to recent literature in order to answer the question: What makes a great quarterback? The results show that the Kestenberg Movement Profile has the potential to aid in the identification of performance enhancing movement qualities. The point is repeatedly made that it can supply professional sports and sports psychology with a more complete and in-depth study of the personality of an athlete.

Levidi, Eleni. *Why And How To Do Dance Therapy With Persons With Borderline Personality Disorder.* Hunter College, 1994.

This thesis answers two questions: why do dance therapy with the borderline personality and how to do dance therapy with the borderline. It is suggested that dance therapy, because of the medium of dance/movement, can be of great therapeutic value for the treatment of borderline personality disorders. Literature on borderline phenomena from several perspectives is reviewed. Emphasis is put on how the psychological development of an identity and a sense of self is based on the following: the organization of body perceptions and motoric actions and the quality of interactions with the early environment. Dance therapy approaches with persons with borderline personality disorder are reviewed. Discussion on dance therapy with borderline personalities focuses on concepts which are viewed as important in formulating a dance/ movement therapy model for working with persons with borderline personality disorder.

Levin, Carrie. *Dance Movement Therapy with Sensory Defensive Children.* Columbia College, 1995.

Approximately five to ten percent of children in this country suffer from some type of sensory integrative dysfunction. The nature of the dysfunction most often leads to difficulty with bonding, serious psychological implications and and poor self-esteem. They typically display behavioral difficulties and have trouble interacting with peers.

Levinbook-Mezamer, Meirav. *Developmental Theory, Object Relations, and Dance/Movement Therapy as Combined References for Therapy with Emotionally Disturbed Children.* Lesley College Graduate School, 1991.

This paper is intended as one link in a lonq chain of works directed toward the uses of body and body movement for therapeutic ends. Psychoanalytically oriented dance-movement therapy is used to identify the specific techniques outlined in this paper. There is an overview of both Developmental Object-Relations theory and the Laban System of Movement Analysis. Two case studies of emotionally disturbed young girls are presented. Clinical application is specifically devoted to putting the theoretical frame of reference to a working test. The final section is a presentation of the personal journey of this writer on the way to becoming a therapist.

Lewis, Gretchen E. *Listen To What They Are Playing: A Learning Experience About Adolescents, Music, and Dance/Movement Therapy.* Antioch/New England Graduate School, 1995.

This thesis will investigate the therapeutic gains made by considering adolescents' preferences for music within a dance/movement therapy session. A review of relevant literature includes an overview of adolescents and music, and a focus on adolescents, music and dance/movement therapy. A self-made questionnaire was sent to every dance/movement therapist registered with the American Dance Therapy Association to access pre-existing views on the importance of adolescents' music preferences. Dance/movement therapists were asked to rate both therapeutic gains and therapeutic challenges which might occur within a dance/movement therapy session where adolescents' music preferences are considered.

Lipschutz, Renee. *Dance Therapy, Movement, and Spirituality: The Exploration and Journey of a Jewish Dance Therapist.* Hunter College, 1988.

This paper is an investigation of the relationship between dance therapy and spirituality. It is a case study based on the writer's personal experience of becoming an observant Jew while studying to become a dance therapist. The role of dance and movement is examined in the Bible, during the Jewish prayer service, Jewish holiday celebrations, the worship of Hasidic Jews, and in Israel. The relationship between Judaism and psychology is investigated, with an emphasis on Jewish mysticism. Analogies are made between concepts in Jewish mysticism and elements of dance therapy and its practice. An Hasidic counseling session is compared with a dance therapy session. In the case study, the author's personal history is presented, leading into a discussion of dance therapy as a spiritual modality and as a means of reaching one's soul.

Lorenz, Coleen H. *The Application of Dance/Movement Therapy in the Treatment of Head Injured Patients.* University of California, Los Angeles, 1992.

The purpose of this study is to explore the effects of dance/movement therapy with the head-injured population. The investigation focuses on how basic mechanisms of recovery, including changes in physical, cognitive, emotional-behavioral, and social domains of functioning, can be addressed and possibly altered by dance/movement treatment interventions. Four head injured subjects are treated with dance/movement therapy for eight weekly sessions. Their clinical courses are documented and discussed in the context of both the head injury and dance/movement therapy literatures. Information gathered for the process descriptions and case study results are subjective both on the part of the subjects and the researcher.

The investigator observed positive changes in two of the four subjects in several areas of functioning. The remaining subjects made little or no progress. Progress differences between the four subjects appeared to be associated with the number of times each client attended the sessions and pre-morbid factors possibly influencing post-injury outcome.

This study has several limitations: 1) the inexperience of the clinician/researcher with this population, 2) the limited number of sessions, 3) the inability to effect multiple domains of functioning within a short-term study, 4) the difficulty generalizing results from a small sample of subjects, and 5) the need to clarify what constitutes progress given the different types of severity of head injury. This pilot study maps possible approaches, methodological issues, and benefits in working with the head injured population. Dance/movement therapy may be efficacious in the rehabilitation of head trauma victims.

Lowery, Tracy. *Dance/Movement Therapy and Assertiveness in African-American Female College Students.* Goucher College, 1992.

The purpose of this study is to determine whether or not levels of assertiveness increased in African-American female college students receiving dance/movement therapy. Literature on assertiveness, the psychology and sociology of women and female college students, the psychology and sociology of African-American women and African-American female college students, and dance/movement therapy are reviewed and integrated.

The study took place at a predominantly African-American university on the East Coast. Eleven African-American female college students were screened for level of assertiveness using the College Self-Expression Scale and a one-to-one interview with this researcher. All of the subjects were selected to participate in the study since nearly all of them expressed an interest in working on their assertiveness skills and some indicated one or more areas in which they felt they could try to be more assertive.

The subjects were randomly divided into an experimental group of five subjects and a control group of six subjects. The experimental group participated in one dance/movement therapy group for 30 minutes but the control group did not. After the session each subject completed the College Self-Expression Scale as a post-measure of assertiveness. Each subject also had a post-interview using the same format as the initial interview. Both interviews were audiotaped. The subjects in both the experimental and the control groups showed an increase in level of assertiveness from pre-test to post-test. However, the overall increase in level of assertiveness for the experimental group was greater than the overall increase for the control group. A two-by-two mixed factor analysis of variance test showed that the increases in levels of assertiveness in both the experimental and the control groups were not statistically significant.

Luca, Khristine. *Identification of Dance/Movement Therapy as a Unique Modality in a Multi-Modal Rehabilitation Center.* Hunter College, 1996.

This research was conducted to measure senior rehabilitation patient's attitudes towards the usefulness of dance/movement therapy as a treatment modality and if they could distinguish the differences and similarities between dance/movement therapy, physical therapy and occupational therapy. The eight (female) and three (male) subjects ranged in age from 66 to 89. The subjects involved in the study were admitted to the Rehabilitation Unit for either hip, wrist, arm, shoulder and/or cervical fractures, cerebral vascular accidents (CVA) or general deconditioning due to previous illness. The subjects were pre-questioned upon admission as to their knowledge of dance/movement, physical, and occupational therapies. They were also asked questions pertaining to their physical, emotional and social well-being. The subject's length of hospitalization was four to five weeks. Most patients participated in three to four dance/movement therapy sessions on average. The data collected from the pre and post-treatment questionnaires were analyzed in two-tiers (Descriptive and Comparative). The findings were positive and proved the author's hypothesis. There were significant increases in the subject's understanding of dance/movement therapy. Subjects could also distinguish this therapy from physical and occupational therapy.

Lucas, Patricia Ann. *The Experience of Evil and Separation From Self: A Dance Movement Therapist's Approach to Working with Problems with Evil.* Naropa Institute, 1992.

The research for this thesis began in studying energetic polarities and their relationship to human pathology. Through dance/movement therapy training, the author was drawn to the view that all existence is energy, looking at herself and others as energetic beings, moving, forming, and communicating through a variety of energetic organizations. There was also recognition that the way we choose to organize our life energy is sometimes out of balance with our environment (either internally within the body or externally in relationship to others). This causes a distorted or blocked flow of energy which we can experience as suffering and disease. An area of study that was of most interest was the relationship between the polarity of Good and Evil and human pathology. The author became curious to better understand what was occurring for clients who reported having problematic experiences of Evil. A significant number of people she worked with during the internship reported feelings of Evil or fears that Evil was going to steal their souls. This provoked a number of questions for me: "What were these people experiencing as Evil? What did they mean when they said Evil? How could I be of service to them? Does Evil really exist?".

Lucier, Constance Frost. *Developmental Play Within the Primary Relationship for Designing Dance/Movement Therapy Intervention.* Goucher College, 1992.

The purpose of this study is to explore the application of play to dance/movement therapy practice. The areas of literature reviewed include: general theories in human developmental processes, the function of play and relationship in those processes, and dance/movement therapy theory and practice. The author correlates the elements of development, relationship, and play to the goals, techniques, and process defined in dance/movement therapy. The researcher's pursuit was to translate how play, within the primary relationship, may serve as a model for therapist intervention in dance/movement therapy.

Three children, paired with their primary caregivers, were recruited from a recreation program, as well as from other contacts. In the selection of mother/child dyads, the researcher ruled out any medical or psychological conditions that might have interfered with the purpose of this study. With the counsel of the children's recreational director, the participants were screened for their capacity to represent the specific developmental stages described in this study and the extent to which the mother and child engaged in a healthy relationship. A set of tasks were designed to structure interactions representative of play and relationship in the developmental process. The mothers selected a task(s) that would best demonstrate their natural relationship and the dyads were videotaped.

Four dance/movement therapy students and professionals whose dance/movement therapy work uses a developmental model were asked to observe the videotape vignettes, and discuss their observations pertaining to the study in context with their own clinical experiences. The participants were encouraged to demonstrate movement interactions related to the discussions. The results of this study are in the form of an edited videotape that alternates takes of: 1) mother/child dyads playing together, and 2) dance/movement therapy students' and professionals' discussions and demonstrations of clinical applications. Meant to serve an educational purpose, the researcher's editing attempts to show the viewer how to apply developmental play in relationship to dance/movement therapy practice. The lack of pathological examples of client development to support the study would suggest future research on this topic.

MacArthur, Leslie. *The Use of Play in Dance/Movement Therapy.* Goucher College, 1992.

The purpose of this study is to examine how dance/movement therapists, working with a variety of populations, perceive play and its role in dance/movement therapy sessions. The writer reviews dance/movement therapy and play literature. The literature reflects the importance of play in normal development and the integral role play has in dance/movement therapy as a means of addressing developmental issues. This research project used an interview format. Ten dance/movement therapists were interviewed in order to determine how they define play, how often they see play in their sessions, where in the session play occurs, and if they use play in working towards population-specific goals.

Results of the interviews revealed that in defining play there were key phrases or ideas common to several of the definitions given by the therapists. Several factors, including the therapist's definition of play, may influence the reported frequency of play in sessions. Other factors include personal theoretical orientation, the population with which the therapist is working, and personal style. This project showed that each therapist interviewed uses play as an intervention and, when appropriate to the group process, facilitates client-initiated play. It was found that the progression of a dance/movement therapy session, and the forms of play reportedly used within each phase of the session, follow a progression similar to that of play in normal development. According to the therapists interviewed, play is most likely to occur during the transition from warm-up to theme development. Play is less likely to occur during warm-up and closure. All therapists interviewed use play to work towards population specific goals.

Maciel, Duan. *An Exploration of a Multi-Modal Creative Arts Therapy Approach to Stewart's Theory of the Archetypal, Affective System in a Psychiatric Institution.* California State University, Hayward, 1996.

The author endeavors to facilitate a creative arts therapy group whose principles of interventions are informed by the affect theory of Louis H. Stewart. Exploration of the core of his work are integrated with techniques of creative arts therapies. Through a description of actual sessions of a therapy group and through a case study of an individual client in this group, the author examines the application of the theory's premises.

Mackay, Fiona K. *Props In Dance/Movement Therapy With ADHD Children.* Goucher College, 1994.

The purpose of this study is to discover which props if any, used during dance/movement therapy sessions are beneficial for working with children diagnosed with Attention Deficit Hyperactivity Disorder (ADHD). The functions of each prop found to be useful and the issues and goals that they address, are discussed in detail. The definition of ADHD, frequency of occurrence, statistics, history, issues, and treatment are discussed. A definition of props and types used with different populations and their function are focused on. Dance/movement therapy, its definition, principles, history, goals, techniques, and interventions are reviewed. These topics were discussed from a broad perspective and specifically in relation to ADHD children and use of props.

Methodology involved interviews with ten registered dance/movement therapists. All of the subjects have been practicing for at least three years and work in both public and private facilities. They all have extensive background in working with children and are familiar with the specific needs and issues of ADHD children. It was found that although many different types of props were used with this population, balls, stretchbands, and parachutes were the most common. This is due to their versatility and their favor with the children. Both the ADHD issues and dance/movement therapy interventions mostly addressed were modulation of energy and affect which is preliminary to subsequent work on other issues. The affect most worked on with props was anger which is an emotion that many ADHD children experience as a result of circumstances created due to their impulsivity, overactivity, and inattention. Other questions examined included props used repeatedly, circumstances which warrant the use of certain props, and memorable experiences regarding the use of props with ADHD children.

The data obtained from the interview questions is organized into charts found in Appendices for quick reference. Salient information is discussed and interpreted.

Majoris, Darcee. *A Self-Exploration of the Importance of Personal Therapy While in Training to be a Dance Therapist.* Hunter College, 1995.

Personal therapy plays an integral part in the training of dance/movement therapists. It facilitates self-exploration that aids dance therapy trainees to be aware of and resolveintrapersonal difficulties that could inhibit their work as therapists. A question arises: How can therapists lead patients on a journey if they have not traveled a similar road themselves?

This thesis focuses on the following: personal therapy and its role in training therapists; content analysis of the author's weekly personal therapy sessions juxtaposed with the author's clinical work in dance therapy; and how personal therapy can aid dance therapy trainees in their clinical work with patients by enhancing their own self-knowledge. The parameters to be analyzed include the author's correlations between issues that arise in her own experience of personal therapy and her clinical work with patients as a dance therapist. The author stresses the importance of being in personal therapy at the same time as training to be a dance therapist and exploring personal patterns of interaction and their relationships to working as a dance therapist.

Maskens, Kathryn E. *The Vision Drive in Ecstasy: A Pilot Study.* Laban Centre for Movement and Dance, 1992.

Masters, Kara. *Rejuvenation Practices of Dance/Movement Therapists in Dealing with Physical and Psychological Job Stress.* University of California, Los Angeles, 1995. (SP)

Matias, Maritza. *Dual Diagnosed Patients and A Dance Therapist's Countertransference: Improving Treatment.* Hunter College, 1993.

The dually diagnosed patient is common in the psychiatric inpatient unit. This thesis focuses on the therapist's awareness of countertransference and its use in improving treatment with this population. The dual diagnosed population will be defined and discussed in terms of diagnostic complications, theories on addiction, treatment modalities, and interventions by dance therapists. Several cases of countertransference reactions will be presented and discussed in the light of the common theories of countertransference and how to handle it in the analytic situation.

Maxwell, Tina A. *Dance Therapy and Verbal Processing-An Effective Combination for the Treatment of Anxiety.* Hunter College, 1993.

This thesis explores the benefits of implementing a dual therapy approach in the treatment of anxiety. Anxiety is primarily defined as a disorder characterized by avoidance. Holistic, psychological, verbal group, and dance therapy literature are explored with relevance to the existing treatment of anxiety. Similarities between dance therapy and mind-body therapies are explored as they both encourage feeling and acting in the here and now. The value of dance therapy and verbal group treatment techniques are supported by existing literature on the use of such combination treatments, as well as examples from practice.

McClanahan, Kristin. *The Language of Movement: A Seven-Month Study of Dance/Movement Therapy With a Severely Retarded Adult.* Antioch/New England Graduate School, 1995.

This paper presents a case study of an institutionalized adult male, and the use of dance/movement therapy as part of his treatment. The purpose of this study is to emphasize the importance of dance/movement therapy as a treatment approach for the mentally retarded population, and suggest that dance/movement therapy can assist this population in moving towards higher levels of functioning. Included in this case study is a review of the literature on the use of dance and other creative arts therapies with those considered developmentally delayed. The case study comprises a history of the client, and an account of weekly individual movement therapy sessions noting the client's process of change over a seven-month period of time; especially the releases of body tension, and an evolution of more spontaneous play initiated by the client.

McFadden, Meredith. *A Literature Review of Relational Development and a Body Image Workshop Design: Intervention into the Mother-Daughter Dyad as Prevention in Pre-Adolescent Girls At-Risk.* Allegheny University of the Health Sciences (formerly Hahnemann University), 1996.

The purpose of this thesis is to address body image issues in girls and women. The identified problem is the prevalence of body image problems among pre-adolescent and adolescent girls and the implications of possessing negative body image. This research consists of a literature review covering a statement of the problem, normative early and adolescent female development, and an overview of family systems theory including a definition of normal family functioning. The review culminates in a design for a body image workshop as prevention for normal pre-adolescent girls who are at-risk and their mothers. There are some prevalent complications in the interpretation of the research data. Most research is conducted on white middle class women and girls. African American and Latina girls and women are often generalized to lower income classes, and often no separation between class and race is acknowledged. Accordingly, results are often skewed. A connection between eating disorders and sexual abuse is recognized in the literature, however it is unfounded because of a lack of research evident in this area. There are inquiries surrounding the current debate within the clinical and research spheres, although there is some question as to why no research has been conducted to draw conclusions.

McGehee, Sharon. *Rhythmical Structure and Duration Experience in the Perception of Environmental Input.* Hunter College, 1980

In order to determine the effect of rhythmical structure on the subjective duration experience and subsequent recognition of patterned sequential stimuli, duration estimates and recognition responses were recorded during the presentation of an audio tape of varying sequences of patterned percussive beats. The independent variables were pattern level and accent placement. Ten subjects listened to a presentation series of six sequence conditions and recorded subjective duration estimates of the intervals of the sequences and were subsequently presented with a recognition series of the same six sequences randomized with nine control sequences for which recognition responses were recorded in a 3 x 2 design. Pattern level was differentially effective on both dependent measures, depending on the presence or absence of account placement. Repeating patterned sequences were judged shorter and recognized better when accent placement was included than when it was not. The results were interpreted to support the supposition that rhythmical patterning of presented sequences of events effectively reduces the subjective duration experience of the presentation interval for those sequences as well as the structural complexity of the sequences. Implications for the diagnosis and treatment of autism were drawn from the hypothesized interaction of rhythmical structure, sequence complexity and duration experience.

McGuire, Liz. *Exploring Shame Through the Use of Movement and Dance.* Hunter College, 1992.

This paper explores the nonverbal expression of shame and its mobilization through the use of movement and dance. Shameful feelings relate to how the self perceives itself; they are by nature emotionally and physically inhibiting to the individual experiencing them. Shame's expression is generally nonverbal since verbalization is difficult due to denial and the overwhelming physiological changes in the body. Blushing and covering one's face to hide from others are indicators of shameful feelings.

The study focuses on the physical expression of shame, particularly the author's movement behaviors associated with these feelings. In order to experience feelings of shame and to observe its manifestation, the author videotaped herself moving and dancing while being observed. Analysis involved corresponding internal-felt sensations and thoughts with observable movement behavior. Feelings of anger and sadness are observed as feelings of shame are experienced. Overcoming the fears of being observed and feeling rejected are at the crux of mobilizing shameful feelings. Changing one's self-concept involves experiencing shame on a body/movement level and allowing the feelings of rejection, anger, sadness and hurt to be felt and integrated into the psyche.

Menzam, Cherionna. *An Authentic Birth: Pre And Perinatal Issues in Authentic Movement.* Naropa Institute, 1996.

In recent years, clinicians have observed that pre and perinatal trauma can be stored in our bodies, apparently as "cellular memory" (Hendricks and Hendricks, 1991), and tends to be recapitulated in our lives (Emerson, 1984). This study investigates the hypothesis that in authentic movement, an expressive movement discipline, traumatic pre and perinatal issues may spontaneously arise in the form of specific types of movement sequences. Videotapes of two authentic movement groups have been analyzed for movement sequences demonstrating pre and perinatal movements and postures previously documented in the field of pre and perinatal psychology and movement therapy.

Movement sequences and postures are described and illustrated, with an intent to serve as guidance for practitioners in identifying pre and perinatal material in their clients' movements.

While a thorough investigation of the effects of authentic movement on the resolution of pre and perinatal trauma is beyond the scope of this thesis, implications for further study and for dance/movement therapy are discussed.

Mesmer, Anne C. *Dance/Movement Therapy, Bereavement and the Family: A Modern Day Ritual.* (SP for alternate route)

This study reports in depth on six sessions conducted with a family (parents and two young children) which had lost the maternal grandmother due to brain cancer. The study integrates and utilizes grief counseling, family systems theory and dance/movement therapy. Main conclusions are: children are effected by grief and often are more in touch with feelings than adults; the ritual of a time, place and framework to deal with these issues is healing; a family has its own process verbally and in movement ; family communication and functioning improves when brought together; bereavement stirs deep feelings that require time for healing.

Mettler, Tricia A. *Dance/Movement Therapy And Self-Concept In Head Injury Rehabilitation.* Antioch/New England Graduate School, 1994.

The purpose of this thesis is to support the hypothesis that dance/movement therapy will help head injured individuals regain more positive, realistic self-concepts. Although head injury affects an individual physically, it also affects him/her psychologically through cognitive, emotional, and social impairments. This thesis will explore dance/movement therapy's role in working experientially to help utilize the physical motion that is available, as well as working with the psychological implications that are manifest in the body. Literature on head injury, dance movement therapy, and self-concept in relation to the gestalt theoretical framework will be reviewed. Also, experiences the author has encountered while working with the head injured population will be discussed.

Miller, Beverly M. *Sacred Sign Dance: A Creative And Therapeutic Integration of Language, Movement, and Spirituality.* Antioch/New England Graduate School, 1992.

This thesis introduces and describes the creation by the author of Sacred Sign Dance, a dance/movement therapy based, creative art form. The motivation and rationale for its development as a therapeutic tool is explored in relation to the following theoretical premise: patriarchy and body-mind dualism in contemporary western society have, to a large degree, oppressed and/or destroyed the innate, empowering consciousness of the human body-mind-spirit trinity and in its place, created a debilitating sense of isolation and indifference or aggression toward ourselves, each other and life in general. To aid in clarifying the proposed reintegrative and healing nature of Sacred Sign Dance, each of its basic components are examined in detail. In addition, Sacred Sign Dance is compared to Eurythmy, other forms of dance/movement therapy, and to the role of shamanic and sacred dance in ancient societies. Responses by witnesses of Sacred Sign Dance presentations are also included to contribute information regarding the effectiveness of Sacred Sign Dance as a vehicle for shared healing and celebration.

Millrod, Eri Tanaka. *Object Relations and Play: Building Houses in Dance/Movement Therapy with Emotionally Disturbed Children.* New York University, 1991.

An exploratory study in which a group of up to five emotionally disturbed children between the ages of 10 and 13 were seen in ten dance/movement therapy sessions over a three week period. The theme for seven out of those ten sessions evolved around temporary houses that the group built and destroyed together. The house building theme is analyzed, using theories of play therapy and object relations, to determine the therapeutic value of using play and objects in play within the dance/movement therapy sessions. It is proposed that play, movement, and dance are the three mediums of expression for children and that all three are equally valuable in children's development. Furthermore, the incorporation of play, movement, and dance by dance/movement therapists in their work with children is particularly recommended for short-term therapy. A survey of dance/movement therapists who have worked or who are working with this population is suggested for further study.

Minott, Danielle Yvonne. *Dance/Movement Therapy In a School Setting in Jamaica: Considerations on the Cross-Cultural Applicability of an American-Based Model.* University of California, Los Angeles, 1992.

There are questions surrounding the cross-cultural applicability of a single dance movement therapy model. This paper explores a dance/movement therapy model utilized at The ERAS Centre, a special education setting in America and the issues around its application in a comparable Jamaican setting, Mico Care Centre. Literature collected from cross-cultural psychology is reviewed including the presentation of information on comparisons of Jamaican and American cultures. The exploration of Jamaican customs and traditions including child rearing practices is made in the context of psychotherapy and its interpersonal implications as carried out within the Jamaican educational environment. The aim is to observe and understand the ramifications of implementing an existing movement therapy model to a new culture. Detailed descriptions of the application of the model as it relates to the student's tolerance of direction, choice, and interaction with the therapist in the therapeutic setting, are presented and illustrated in sessions with four boys, two from each culture. The conclusion discusses the significance of the evidence for dance/movement therapy as a model of therapeutic intervention.

Moncrieff, Mary. *The Relationship Between Dance Symbols and Group Process in a Dance Therapy Session.* Hunter College, 1985.

This thesis is a study of the relationship between symbolism and group process in dance therapy. It involves a structural analysis of movement and verbal behavior contained in a group dance therapy session. This structural analysis serves as a means of interpreting group dance symbols in terms of group process theory. The major topics addressed in this study are structural development of the session and how it gives rise to the dance symbol, the development of the session as it reflects the group process, and the dance symbol as it supports this process.

The dance symbols within this session follow a developmental progression from lower to higher levels of complexity. Each of these levels contains symbolic content unique to its own level. The development of the session is reflected in the building and diminishing aspects of these levels. The layers of dance symbols are seen as a symbolic representation of the growth and development of the group. The entire session is seen as one symbolic dance: a dance about group members rediscovering themselves as individuals, gathering themselves into a group, interacting, performing together and assuming new and healthier identities.

Moogan, Linden. *The Effects of a Nine Session Dance/Movement Therapy Program Tailored for a Mentally Retarded Teenager Using the Person Centered Planning Approach.* Hunter College, 1996.

The purpose of this study is to explore behavioral change over time in a severely retarded individual in dance/movement therapy treatment. Behavioral categories were identified to follow throughout the course of treatment. In order to develop a behavioral objective assessment for the subject, 'A Personal Profile' derived from the Person-Centering Planning approach (Mount, 1992) was tailored to the subject for the purpose of formulating an intervention strategy. The subject's progress was then subjectively rated on the basis of written observations, conferences with the subject's mother, and conferences with co-leaders/instructors. For the purpose of this study, body movement was a central focus. The method of observation used in assessing the subject's behavior was derived from Laban's system of movement analysis. Interactive evaluative structures are related to the Maraschach Interactive Methods (MIM). The results of this study indicate that dance/movement therapy treatment was used successfully to reduce emotional withdrawal and promote communication skills in the subject.

Moore, Christine Ann. *A Naturalistic Study of Intergenerational Movement Patterns Between Three Generations of Women.* Allegheny University of the Health Sciences formerly Hahnemann University), 1993.

Literature on intergenerational transmission assumes that numerous variables are transmitted through generations of a family. Intergenerational research, however, lacks empirical data to validate this process. Research and theories have identified the importance of the woman's role in the intergenerational process. This study was designed to investigate whether intergenerational transmission process of a family can be directly observed through the family's nonverbal behavior. It specifically focuses on the nonverbal behavior of a grandmother, mother, and daughter from one family to determine if there were any similarities in their movement style. The hypothesis of this study stated that similarities will be observed between the three women's use of phrasing and that the number of similarities will vary between the different dyads. Results partially supported the study's hypothesis. Findings indicated some similarities between the three women's use of phrasing. Several similarities were found between two generations of women, mostly between the mother and daughter. Results are inconclusive due to low inter-observer reliability and other limitations of this study. However, the implications and importance for future studies in understanding the intergenerational process through movement is clearly illustrated.

Moore, Melissa. *Dance/Movement Therapy with Physically and Sexually Abused Children.* University of California, Los Angeles, 1993.(SP)

Moorman, Lawaune. *Realistic Goals for Short-Term Hospitalized Psychotic Females: A Dance/Movement Therapy Survey.* Columbia College, 1986. (C-Vol.I)

Morningstar, Dawn. *The Development of the Movement Analysis Toward the Identification of Movement Characteristics of Male Adolescent Sexual Offenders.* Allegheny University of the Health Sciences (formerly Hahnemann University), 1993.

There are 18,100 juveniles arrested for a sexual offense per year (U.S. Dept. of Commerce) but the research on adolescent sexual offense is minimal (Wyatt, 1988). To date, no literature contains research on the nonverbal behaviors of male adolescent sexual offenders and there seems to be no single profile of the typical sexual offender. This pilot study is designed to assess differences between male adolescent sexual offenders and male adolescents never accused of a sexual offense. Each of the ten subjects was videotaped in a seated verbal interview and asked questions about themselves such as likes and dislikes and goals for the future. Two raters observed videotapes of the subjects and completed a movement scale compiled by the researcher. A Kappa statistic was performed on each group to assess interrater reliability for each item. Body attitude, integrated posture-gesture mergers (Lamb, 1973) and dominance/submissive displays received moderate to substantial Kappa agreement. The hypothesis that there would be differences seen in body attitude, use of effort, phrasing, interactional components and rhythmic alterations of tension-flow was somewhat substantiated.

Moroney, Tracy. *The Implications of Using Rhythmic Circle Formations in the Treatment of Adult Schizophrenic Patients.* University of California, Los Angeles, 1996. (SP)

Morris, Catherine B. *From Intern To Therapist: A Personal Account of Movement Therapy As An Important Intervention With Brain Injured And Stroke Patients.* Lesley College Graduate School, 1991.

This study presents a personal perspective on the use of movement therapy and supports it as an important component for the healing process for recovering brain injured and stroke patients. The setting for this study is a rehabilitation hospital in the Boston area. An introductory personal statement is made based on the creative process of writing as guided by the clinical experience as well as a general overview of dance/movement therapy in rehabilitation.

Four clinical case studies are documented as well as a movement therapy group that provides information on the components of the therapeutic process through dance therapy. Supervision and countertransference in relation to the effectiveness of treatment are examined. The personal process of training as an intern to becoming a therapist is discussed.

Morrissee, Christine Marie. *The Impact of Intergenerational Movement Therapy on Interactional and Engagement Behaviors in a Geriatric Population.* Allegheny University of the Health Sciences (formerly Hahnemann University), 1994.

This study is based on the hypothesis that residents of a nursing home will demonstrate more behavior of interaction and engagement during intergenerational dance/movement therapy sessions than during geriatric dance/movement therapy as measured by a movement parameters scale and a nurses' questionnaire. This study was undertaken to provide research on what types of treatment are most effective with long-term residents of a geriatric facility in the development and maintenance of social interactions and other previously acquired skills. Through the sustainment of interpersonal relationships, the overdependence and deterioration of the residents' psychosocial state can be delayed.

This study examines effects on the elderly alone. This study ran for four consecutive weeks and consisted of seven subjects. They received geriatric dance/movement therapy every other week for approximately one hour and intergenerational dance/movement therapy with children aged four years from a local child development center for one hour every other week. All groups were videotaped and rated by dance/movement therapy students. In addition, nurses filled out questionnaires after every session concerning the residents' social behaviors. The findings of this pilot study supported the hypothesis that interaction parameters increased when the elderly engaged in intergenerational dance/movement therapy. It was also demonstrated that the geriatrics' social attitudes improved slightly during the rest of the day of intergenerational dance/movement therapy treatment as reflected in the mean scores of the nurses' evaluations. No significant values could be determined, however, as sample size was too small.

Morton, Patricia. *A Transgenerational Approach to Addictive Behavior: Movement Psychotherapy as an Intervention.* Hunter College, 1993.

This paper proposes that the rigid all or none coping mechanism and behaviors of addicts may be viewed psycho-developmentally. This perspective considers the impact of a transgenerational, unempathetic caretaking environment on the life of parents with addictions. Addictive "acting out", ritualized behaviors can be seen as dependency on the intense, cyclical emotional extremes of gambling, relationships, food, sex, work, drugs and alcohol.

A case study of a twenty year old female in recovery for food and alcohol addictions is presented. Nine movement psychotherapy sessions offered her opportunities to explore alternatives to her rigid, ritualized behaviors. At the conclusion of the nine sessions she increased her flexibility by acknowledging, accepting and moving through her denial, grandiosity, shame, control issues and anger, which were the triggers for her addictive acting out behaviors.

Moskow, Jill. *Dance Therapy as an Intervention in Breast Cancer Patients.* Hunter College, 1996.

This thesis is an exploration of dance/movement therapy as a treatment modality for the psychological effects of breast cancer on women. The literature review focuses on the ways women cope with diagnosis and medical treatment of breast cancer; the coping strategies these patients utilize; the interventions commonly used to aid in coping; and how dance/movement therapy is a beneficial modality for intervention.

The methodology of the study was a pre-test/post-test, preexperimental design. The patients were assessed with a body image scale and a set of phenomenological questions prior to and following six weeks of dance/movement therapy sessions. The results suggest that dance/movement therapy helped patients to integrate their body images and issues regarding socialization.

Moyer Holmberg, Mimi. *Change in Leadership Study Concerning the Dance Movement Therapy Department and the Impact of this Change on the Graduate Classes of 1989 and 1990.* Hunter College, 1994.

This thesis examines the impact—disequilibrium/equilibrium—on the system containing the dance therapy graduate students classes of 1989 and 1990 after change in leadership of the Dance Therapy Program at Hunter College. An analysis was performed on quantifiable (numerical) and qualitative (descriptive words/phrases) data obtained from a study of graphs and questionnaires distributed to both the first ('90) and second ('89) year graduate students (respondents) of dance therapy.

The results of the data were summarized on three tables evaluating: 1) Emotional response; 2) Student/teacher relationship; and 3) Response to Program Elements in respect to both past and new leaders for both class groups. The hypothesis was confirmed that a disequilibrium would occur immediately following the change in leadership, and that over time, equilibrium (balance) would be restored within the system.

Musacchio, Jean. *The Great Female Cover-up: Denial of Envy and Competition Between Women; Its implications for Dance/Movement Therapy.* Hunter College, 1992.

Envy, jealousy, and competition between women have long been tabooed topics. In this thesis, the relevant literature on the development of women's relationships and these particular obstacles to their growth is explored. A major premise of this thesis is that since the majority of dance/movement therapists are women, this investigation of female envy and competition is pertinent to the field of dance/movement therapy; it has relevance to both the fledgling therapist as she goes through the socialization process of a dance/movement therapy training program as well as the more experienced, professional dance/movement therapist as she seeks the support and solace of other women colleagues.

Suggestions are made as to how the Hunter College Dance/Movement Therapy Master's Program might modify both didactic and experiential coursework to bring attention to women's denial of the envy and competition between them. Finally, it is recommended that the typical female-female relationship of supervisor-supervisee can only be fully understood with these covert aspects to women's relationships in mind. Envy, jealousy, and competition between women should be brought into the light where they can be examined, shared, and recognized as part of women's wanting.

Nace, Frieda. *People, Problems and Possibilities: Dance/Movement Therapy—Moving Toward Wholeness From Infancy to Old Age. A Public Access Cable Television Production.* Antioch/New England Graduate School, 1990.

The need for greater publicity and marketing of dance/movement therapy has been designated by an American Dance Therapy Association membership poll as one of the top priorities of the national organization. In an effort to address this need, a one-hour program was produced on the local public-access cable television station introducing dance/movement therapy to the general community. In a talk-show format, seven dance/movement therapists were interviewed, three of them demonstrating their work with film clips from actual dance/movement therapy sessions. Accompanying a video-taped copy of the one-hour program is a written thesis which outlines the background of the project, discusses the significance of this type of publicity to the field, and includes the outline and pre-scripts for the show, as well as a summary and discussion of the project.

Nadvornik, Kristi Anne. *Anxiety In Leadership: An Investigation of a Dance Therapy Intern's Anxious Movements and the Underlying Causes.* Hunter College, 1988.

A comparison of leadership and non-leadership situations was done in order to discover the relationship between anxious movements and a leadership role. The review of literature includes definitions and origins of anxiety, five prominent psychological theories of anxiety, and anxiety in leadership. Four videotapes were used in the selection of four movements that characterize anxiety in the author. Three of these tapes were dance/movement therapy sessions in which the author was the leader and the fourth was a movement improvisation. Two raters recorded the number of anxious movements present in six random ten second segments of the control tape (the movement improvisation) and the anxiety tape. An analysis of the data revealed significant differences indicating an association between the two tapes and the number of anxious movements recorded. An examination of the issues arising at the time the anxious movements occurred discusses the possible underlying causes of the anxious movements and feelings concerning the issues.

Nagy, Idilko. *The Therapeutic Mechanism of Ritual Dances and Dance Therapy.* Hunter College, 1996.

This is a theoretical paper that compares the common healing factors in shamanistic or ritual dances and dance therapy. It focuses on three elements of the healing processes, rhythm, group involvement, and symbolism, and suggests a "new" therapeutic factor, altered states of consciousness (trance). Finally biochemical processes and emotional correlations are discussed, emphasizing the role of endorphins as a therapeutic mechanism.

Nast-Brandt, Nava. *Creative Art Therapies and Multiple Personality Disorder.* Naropa Institute, 1993.

The assumption of this thesis is that MPD treatment as a whole can be furthered by the inclusion of art, movement and sandplay therapy. Communication within the system, specifically between host and alters, can be enhanced through the creative modalities using non-verbal and symbolic modes. Improved communication can increase cooperation and facilitate more rapid integration.

Neglia, Nicole A. *The Problem of Health Care Delivery for Haitian Americans and It's Implications for Dance Therapy.* Hunter College, 1988.

This paper includes a literature review that covers the history of the Haitian people and the development of their "personality" and cultural behavior. The influence of African culture and religion on their world view is discussed. The importance of Voodoo, an indigenous combination of African Vodun and French Catholicism is explored. Haitian theories of illnesses revolve around spiritual and natural causes. Pressures of acculturation, added to individual and cultural factors, lead to unique problems for the Haitian American immigrant receiving health care. Specific problems to be aware of are: language difficulties, immigration status, attitudes towards authority, shame about illness, fear of hospitalization and racial discrimination.

The case study follows the seven sessions of treatment of a middle class Haitian American wife in a private psychiatric setting. Treatment was not as effective as it might have been because cultural assumptions were made about both her symptoms and her family relationships. Treatment recommendations call for an improved awareness of the health care provider's own cultural biases as well as awareness of Haitian American attitudes. Studies show that this increased knowledge improves delivery of health care and leads to more effective treatment. Other recommendations include a more direct approach in counseling and the use of older, respected family and/or community members for support. Dance therapy fits into the mental health care of Haitian Americans quite well because of positive cultural attitudes towards dance. Dance is seen as a sign of well being. Dance therapists should be aware of Haitian American movement patterns.

Nemetz, Laurice D. European. *Balkan. and Middle Eastern Folk Dance and its use in Dance/Movement Therapy.* Goucher College, 1993.

The author explores how folk dance forms can be used today in the field of dance/movement therapy. The author traces the history and theories of dance/movement therapy, starting with the roots of modern dance, and then outlining developmental theory. Next, the author examines the history of folk dance, focusing on rhythms, patterns, and social roles. In an integrative chapter, the author explains folk dance forms and their relationship to dance/movement therapy. Charts are provided to clearly outline some examples and their use as a dance/movement therapy intervention.

A video tape was created to accompany the project and to emphasize visually how folk dance can be integrated into the dance/movement therapy process. The video follows the work of the thesis closely. In addition to a brief history, several of the developmental stages are demonstrated in movement, and applicable folk dances are also shown. The video focuses on applications of using folk dance in dance/movement therapy concentrating on rhythm, patterns and social roles.

In the final discussion, three main areas are addressed: implications of this project, use of folk dance as an assessment device, and using folk dance as an educational tool. It focuses on the idea that developmental theory can be related to the overall maturation process of humanity. Just as movement characteristics indicate a developmental stage, the changes in folk dances reflect an overall growth in humankind's evolution. Folk dance forms, which represent primarily the symbiotic stage, can be used to rework early stages of development, as well as being a useful assessment tool. Since the basic forms of folk dance are accessible regardless of a dancer's skill, folk dance can also be a powerful and effective means to introduce the concepts of dance/movement therapy.

Neriya, Pallavi Pai. *Supervision in Dance Movement Therapy: Students and Supervisors Perspectives.* Goucher College, 1991.

This is an interview-based study of clinical supervision in dance/movement therapy. It attempts to provide students, supervisors, and educators, a better understanding of this important aspect of dance/movement therapy training. The hope is to enhance professional and personal learning through the supervision structure.

The review of literature is a) psychotherapy and creative arts therapies and training in these fields; b) history, principles, process and training in dance/movement therapy specifically in the Goucher College Graduate Dance/Movement Therapy program; c) clinical supervision in psychotherapy; d) integrated material on clinical supervision in dance/movement therapy.

Nine students and six supervisors of the Goucher College Graduate Dance/Movement Therapy program were the sample population. Of the nine students, three were second-year students who had just completed their first-year training, three were continuing students who had just completed their second-year course work and were enrolled for an extra semester to complete their thesis, and three were recent graduates who had just completed the entire training program. The subjects were interviewed on their experience of feedback, format, expectations and perspectives within their supervision structures.

The interviews reveal that students and supervisors prefer receiving and providing feedback in a manner that is gentle, straightforward, non-judgmental and constructive. The research reveals several techniques of supervision which include discussions of groups, reviewing videotaped therapy sessions, and using experiential and role-playing techniques and creative movement sessions. The interviews reveal that most students and supervisors would like supervision two hours a week, especially in the second year. Students reported having no specific expectations of supervision in the first year, but they were very aware and had specific agendas as to what they wanted to get out of the second-year supervision experience. Students and supervisors both expected that students should come into supervision with enthusiasm, curiosity, a commitment to learn, and a realistic assessment of their skills and knowledge. The ideal supervision relationship was one that allowed an open dialogue between student and supervisor. All students and supervisors differentiated between supervision and therapy and stated that although the skills for each might run parallel, the goals were different. The interviews also revealed suggestions for creating different formats for evaluation.

Future research in this area could further support and expand this study by including views and suggestions from supervisors and students from programs outside Goucher.

Nieman, Margaret Snider. *The Function of Touch in Two Dance Therapy Sessions.* Hunter College, 1984.

How touch functions in dance therapy was studied. Some authors believe that touch in therapy can only be sexual. This study's hypothesis was that touch would occur more often during issues such as support, nurturance, and closeness, than during sexuality and aggression. Two dance therapy sessions with forensic patients were videotaped and the movement before, during and after there was touch was analyzed. Touch appeared to function in nine ways: for play, support, communication, closeness, guidance and helping, nurturance, discipline and control, to facilitate group interaction, and to infantilize.

Nixon, Anne. *The Integration of Dance/Movement Theapy and Dramatic Structure Techniques with Violent Adolescents.* University of California, Los Angeles, 1995. (SP)

Noble, Eileen A. *Dance/Movement Therapy and the Hyperactive Child.* University of California, Los Angeles, 1992.

This is a case study that includes both clinical observations and a relatively objective means of monitoring the child's psychological and behavioral states following dance/movement therapy. The author's eclectic client-centered approach to the problem of attention deficit hyperactivity disorder incorporates therapeutic interventions that may promote relaxation, emotional release, and physical self-control by means of body focusing, covert rehearsal, muscle tension/relaxation techniques, imagery, and enactment of past scenes. Through statistical analysis, it was found that symptoms initially decreased and then increased over time when a comparison was done between hyperactivity factors, classroom raters, and dance/movement therapy. It is suggested a longitudinal study be developed.

Noel, L. Gwen. *Illness as Teacher: A Dance Therapy Approach to Cancer and Other Serious Illness.* Naropa Institute, 1995.

The purpose of this paper is to investigate and discuss the concept of body/mind healing as defined in selected references, identify the principles common to all three and integrate these ideas into a professional approach to dance/movement psychotherapy as applied to individuals diagnosed with cancer or other chronic illnesses. The primary references are: "The Process of Healing in Dance/Movement Therapy", a paper by Christine Caldwell, MA ADTR; *The Four Fold Way:* Walking the Paths of the Warrior, Teacher, Healer, and Visionary, by Angeles Arrien, Ph.D.; and *The Healing Forces of Music*, by Randall McClellan, Ph.D.

Norman, Victoria. *Dance/Movement Therapy: Professional Development Through Publication*. Goucher College, 1993.

The purpose of this study is to elucidate book and journal publishing, the publication process, the history of publication in dance/movement therapy and to gather recommendations from published dance/movement therapists and publishing professionals, in order to determine the appropriate resources and procedures necessary for publication of dance/movement therapy manuscripts.

A literature review of a) journal and book publishing practices; b) procedures for the publication of articles and books; and c) the history and development of publication in the dance/movement therapy profession is presented.

Five dance/movement therapists with experience as authors and five publishing professionals were recruited to participate in the study. The interview questions were designed by this researcher to elicit recommendations for the publication of dance/movement therapy articles and books. The subjects' audiotaped responses to the interview questions were transcribed and are summarized and reported.

There is a discussion of the data collected on the procedures and resources for publication of dance/movement therapy manuscripts. The implications of the results indicate that successful publication requires an educated and professional approach; that established practices for the publication of professional manuscripts are universal and appropriate for dance/movement therapists; and that there are issues unique to the dance/movement therapy profession that effect writing and publication.

Although limited to a small number of views, a high rate of agreement is shown regarding publication procedures and resources even though there was a great deal of diversity and experience among the subjects. Dance/movement therapy research, because it is new and innovative, is recommended as a rich source of material for publication and may be regarded as particularly appealing to journal editors and book publishers.

North, Carol J. *Investigating the Mind-Body Relationship: The Psychological and Physical Effects of Developmental Dance/Movement Therapy on a Five Year Old Nonverbal Child with Autism*. California State University, Hayward, 1995.

A dance/movement therapy model utilizing sensory-motor interventions and object relations theory was created and used with a five year old nonverbal child with autism. A complete review of the autistic disorder is provided along with relevant developmental dance/movement therapy literature. The study consisted of three months of twice a week therapy. Physical effects were measured by the Peabody Developmental Motor Scales(Folio and Fewell, 1983) both before and after the three months of treatment. Psychological effects were measured by frequency rating of selected variables known to be associated with autism such as reciprocal social interactions, direct eye contact, subject initiated movement and synchrony with investigator. It is hypothesized that nonverbal communications are reflective of psychological state. It was also hypothesized that the body awareness emphasis of dance/movement therapy would remediate physical coordination and facilitate gross motor progress. Using the measures employed, the subject did evidence improvement in gross motor skills and social interaction.

O'Reilly, Elaine M. *Dancing In The Mirror: An Autobiographical Narrative*.
Antioch/New England Graduate School, 1996.

The application of dance/movement therapy is examined. An in-depth view of a patient's experiences while participating in an outpatient psychiatric program and the simultaneous experiences of a dance/movement therapist in training are presented. Movement sessions are described in detail and emphasize the process of healing through engagement with one's body, connection with other people, and the discovery of the power within that aids in reframing past negative experiences. The movement sessions are categorized into three specific phases, the initiation, working, and transformation phase. These phases apply to the healing process of a patient and a dance/movement therapist in training and are examined within the Stone Center's self-in-relation model. The parallels are highlighted with an exploration of the countertransference process. Finally, the transformation phase concludes the work of the patient and trainee, and emphasizes the effectiveness of dance/movement therapy.

O'Toole, Barbara. *The Movement Psychodiagnostic Inventory and the Luria-Neuropsychological Battery: A Theoretical Foundation for Empirical Research in Psychopathology.* Allegheny University of the Health Sciences (formerly Hahnemann University), 1993.

This study addresses the problem of inadequately stated scientific bases for the assumptions of movement analysis. The purpose of this study is to: 1) develop theoretical bases for inquiry into neurological dysfunctioning and psychological distress manifested in movement behaviors, 2) to investigate neurological behavior in relation to functional and expressive movement, 3) to establish a rationale for combining the Davis' Movement Psychodiagnostic Inventory (1990) and the Luria-Nebraska Neuropsychological Battery (1980) for the purpose of psychological testing. This study examines if the appraisal of movement as observable manifestations of inner states can be correlated with neuropsychological testing for external validation. The goal of this study includes a correlation research design for the comparative examination of diagnostic movement assessment and neuropsychological testing of functioning as it is related to psychological and behavioral dysfunctioning.

Oglesby, Taysha K. *A Holistic View of the Development of the Hunter College Dance/Movement Therapy Program.* Hunter College, 1996.

This study compiles the perceptions toward the Hunter College Dance/Movement Therapy Program of the internship supervisors and the students of the program's first two graduating classes. The methodology consisted of researching preliminary background material and the distribution of surveys to the classes. Of eight surveys, which were sent to the internship supervisors who comprised the accessible population, four were returned. Of the sixteen surveys sent to the accessible population of the students, nine were returned. This compilation presents a holistic view of the initial stages of the Hunter College Dance/Movement Therapy Program.

Ojala, Emily. *Dance/Movement Therapy With a Developmentally Disabled Adolescent Utilizing The Kestenberg Movement Profile.* Antioch/New England Graduate School, 1995.

Dance/movement therapy (DMT) utilizing the Kestenberg Movement Profile (KMP) as an assessment tool and as a theoretical and developmental framework is presented in this case study of a developmentally disabled adolescent. Literature on the use of psychotherapy with the developmentally disabled is discussed and applied to DMT and the KMP. Results and analysis of the subject's KMP are presented and treatment goals are formed based on the findings. Questions are raised and discussed such as the value of constructing a KMP versus simply using one's training in the KMP for assessment and forming treatment goals. Finally, recommendations for further research are given.

Olsen, Janet. *Dance/Movement Therapy in Day-Care Centers: An Implementation Based on Erikson's Developmental Stages.* Hunter College, 1992.

The purpose of this thesis is to examine how dance/movement therapy benefits children in daycare centers. Day-care literature is reviewed and the pros and cons of day-care versus home-reared children in terms of child development are discussed. Erik Erikson's developmental stages provide a foundation on which to build a theoretical program involving dance/movement therapy in day-care. Finally, a plan implementing dance/movement therapy in existing day-care programs is provided along with exercises for each of Erikson's stages from birth to six years of age.

Omeragic-Mestanagic, Gordana. *Transferences and Countertransference in Dance Movement Therapy: A Case Study of an Eight Year Old Child with Emotional and Behavioral Problems.* Laban Centre for Movement and Dance, 1992.

Orth, Carol. *The Career Choice of Dance/Movement Therapy: A Reflection of Personality and Development.* Goucher College, 1993.

The purpose of this study is to develop a perspective on the past and present influences in one's life which lead to entering the field of dance/movement therapy. A literature review of theories of personality and career choice, as supported by the evolution of psychological thought, precedes a fuller discussion of dance/movement therapy. A review of four of the pioneers of dance/movement therapy, their personalities and their professional development is included along with the principles and goals of dance/movement therapy. An integration of the theories of personality and career choiceis applied to the pioneers in order to better understand the process of selecting dance/movement therapy as a career.

A study, which was conducted through the use of the Myers-Briggs Type Indicator (MBTI) and survey responses, explored the backgrounds and personality traits of dance/movement therapists. This study projected that dance/movement therapists endeavor to emulate the spirit of the early pioneers which resulted from a combination of intuitive and feeling preferences, the very catalyst to their pursuit of dance/movement therapy.

One hundred forty-seven Academy of Dance Therapists, Registered (ADTR) were randomly selected from the American Dance Therapy Association (ADTA) Registry. Each subject was sent an MBTI and questionnaire with a letter of explanation inviting participation along with a pre-addressed stamped envelope. Thirty-four or twenty-four percent of subjects responded. The results obtained in this study indicated that a majority of dance/movement therapists in this representative sample possess intuitive and feeling preferences. Additionally, the results indicated that a proportionate number of dance/movement therapists were involved in some form of dance prior to entering the field, indicating a development into the choice of dance/movement therapy as a career.

Papastratigaki, Maria. *Humour in Mirroring.* Laban Centre for Movement and Dance, 1994.

Papillon, S.A. *Case Study of a 28 year Old Paranoid Schizophrenic Male.* Hunter College, 1976.

Parasuram, Kala. *Techniques Used in Dance/Movement Therapy with Cerebral Palsied Adolescents.* Goucher College, 1992.

The purpose of this study is to examine the use of the dance/movement therapy techniques of mirroring, music, voice and props with cerebral palsied adolescents. Three male adolescents with cerebral palsy were the subjects of this study. The researcher conducted eight weekly individual dance/movement therapy sessions with the subjects. The results of this work are documented in the form of case studies presenting the researcher's process notes which include details on the dynamics of the session with a focus on the techniques that were used, the rationale for the introduction of the same and the subject's response to them. In the overall analyses, it was observed that the use of mirroring helped to increase participation, initiation and focus; the use of voice helped to increase body part awareness and expressive movement; the use of props helped to increase expression of affect and movement range; and the use of music helped to increase motivation and participation. It was also observed that each technique was specifically useful to address an area of adolescent issues. Mirroring addressed self-identity and selfhood, voice addressed body awareness and body image, props addressed expression of feelings and music addressed social issues.

Parland, Nancy Marie. *The Creative Process In a Dance/Movement Therapy Session With Patients With Alzheimer's Disease.* Antioch/New England Graduate School, 1996.

Alzheimer's disease is a dementing illness that effects many of the elderly in our society. Dance/movement therapy is a psychotherapy that utilizes the body and elements of dance to enable people to explore and express their inner world and thus provide better quality of life. This thesis will explore the process of developing and implementing a dance/movement therapy group with the patients on an Alzheimer's unit of an inpatient hospital. I have chosen the heuristic method of research which is a method that involves total immersion in the subject being investigated. Included will be subjective data gathered from the author's experiences, as well as a thorough examination of Alzheimer's disease and information concerning methods and experiences other dance/movement therapists have explored in working with this population. By reporting the results in a heuristic manner, it is hoped it provides a better understanding of the actual process of planning and implementing a dance/movement therapy group with this population. There is also the possibility that these ideas are universal to the process of leading dance/movement therapy groups with any population.

Parr, Susan. *Moving Bodies of Water.* Lesley College Graduate School, 1996.

This thesis is an exploration of the healing and discovery process of dance movement therapy in water. Heuristic research is used to look at the author's history and relationship with water and movement. Movement in the water is used as a personal therapeutic modality, and the author shares her process, insights and growth.

Case study methodology is used to look at four sessions of dance movement therapy in water with a teen parent, and a six week dance movement therapy group in water with people with HIV/AIDS. A questionnaire and individual interviews are used. Dance and movement, water, dreams, countertransference issues, mask making, writing and photography are used as expressive therapy techniques. Documentation of these artistic modalities is included.

Parra, Lisa. *Role of Culture in Understanding Behavior and Transferential Reactions of Hispanic Children in Dance/Movement Therapy Context.* University of California, Los Angeles, 1996. (SP)

Parry, Annie E. *Dance Therapy/Authentic Movement and the Encounter with the Inner Child.* Laban Centre for Movement and Dance, 1995.

Perea, Paulina Eva. *Using Ceremony in Dance Therapy.* Naropa Institute, 1991.

This paper is written in two parts. The first is a description of the three kingdoms: plant, animal and mineral, and the four elements: earth, air, fire, and water, and the symbols (primarily Native

American) of healing that are inherent to them. The second part is how to connect to these symbols of healing in dance therapy.

Pereira-Stubbs, Filipa. *The Use of Rhythm in Dance Movement Therapy: A Critical Review of the Literature.* Laban Centre for Movement and Dance, 1994.

Perrin, Anne Marie. *Dance Therapy with Borderline Personality Disordered Patients.* Hunter College, 1992.

This thesis examines dance therapy techniques used with borderline personality disordered patients beginning with a definition of borderline patients which includes common clinical features and commonly employed defense mechanisms. Developmental theory is discussed as it relates to the etiology of borderline character formation. Verbal treatment techniques and dance therapy techniques are reviewed and a discussion of which best facilitates treatment of the borderline patient.

Peterson, Kirsten Marie. *Short-Term Dance/Movement Therapy with Emotionally Disturbed Adolescents.* Goucher College, 1991.

The purpose of this study is to document and explore the issues/themes/affect that appear in dance/movement therapy group sessions conducted with emotionally disturbed adolescents in a short-term psychiatric setting. The dance/movement therapy goals, interventions, and techniques formulated and used to address these issues/themes/affect are recorded and discussed. The literature review discusses dance/movement therapy, crisis intervention, short-term (brief) psychodynamic therapy, and in-patient group therapy. "Normal" adolescent development, emotional disturbance in adolescence, and psychotherapy with adolescents is addressed. An integrative chapter discusses short-term adolescent group psychotherapy, short-term dance/movement therapy, and dance/movement therapy with emotionally disturbed adolescents. Dance/movement therapy is assumed to be an effective modality for the treatment of emotionally disturbed adolescents in a short-term psychiatric setting.

For nine weeks this writer/therapist conducted and followed the process of three sections of dance/movement therapy groups for a total of 16 sessions per section. Immediately after each session, the process of the dance/movement therapy groups were recorded following a process note guideline. This guideline facilitated the observation and recording of the occurrence of group issues/themes/affect, movement, interaction, interventions and techniques used and the goal/outcome of the dance/movement therapy session. The issues/themes/affect were organized into three categories corresponding to a) body/self awareness; b) self-expression; and c) interpersonal relationships. Clinical case vignettes are presented to illustrate the patterns of occurrence, connections between group membership and context of the group, specific goals formulated to foster a working through of the issues/themes/affect, and the dance/movement therapy interventions and techniques used to facilitate the group process. The relationship between short-term dance/movement therapy with emotionally disturbed adolescents and the issues/themes/affect that appear during group dance/movement therapy sessions are discussed. The characteristics of short-term group dance/movement therapy with emotionally disturbed adolescents including specific interventions and techniques, the process, the therapist's role, group composition and transference-countertransference issues are also discussed.

Phipps, Kelly M. *A Place For My Self: Issues of Space in Dance/Movement Therapy with Women in a Homeless Shelter.* Allegheny University of the Health Sciences (formerly Hahnemann University), 1995.

As homelessness in the United States continues to rise, research into the specific needs for treatment of this population is increasing. Both personal and social factors contribute to homelessness as well as different reasons due to gender (North and Smith, 1993). Loss of personal, interpersonal and societal space occur as a result of homelessness. This loss of spatial boundaries can lead to the inability of an individual to overcome his homeless condition. This study was undertaken in an effort to demonstrate a relationship between issues of space among the homeless and dance/movement therapy concepts, to produce a program that would be beneficial to women living in a homeless shelter. As literature pertaining to dance/movement therapy with the homeless is extremely limited, the study consisted of a literature review of women and homelessness, space and dance/movement therapy with relevant populations. In addition, clinical application of dance/movement therapy to this population is given and illustrated with short case vignettes. Findings showed that dance/movement therapy concepts of space were applicable to traumas such as physical and sexual abuse, drug addiction and victimization experience by homeless women. The non-verbal nature and use of the body in dance/movement therapy is able to address these issues at the site of their experience. The conclusion is that dance/movement therapy, especially work geared toward personal space and boundary development, can play a beneficial role in helping women escape patterns of homelessness.

Plattner, Michele. *Personal Process Integrated into the Therapist Training—An Aspect of Experiential Learning.* Naropa Institute, 1990.

This thesis explores how the trainee's personal issues, patterns, and experiences can become an integrated part of his/her therapist training. In the review of literature, experiential approaches to therapist training are discussed. A survey, conducted among students and graduates of the dance/movement therapy program at The Naropa Institute, inquired about the participants' experiences with the Therapist Training Cycle which is an educational paradigm used to train therapist skills.

Along with a new definition of personal process as an integrated part in therapist training, this survey has provided valuable documentation of students' experiences in a process oriented training setting.

Press, Estelle. *A Reichian Approach to Dance Therapy.* Hunter College, 1982.

This paper integrates the work of dance therapy as developed by Marion Chace with the character analytic and bioenergetic discoveries and techniques of Wilhelm Reich. Dance therapy is a recent development in the field of psychotherapy. As our field expands professionally, the need for more concrete and systematic theory and goals increases. Dance therapists must be able to substantiate their work. The therapeutic process in dance therapy focuses on the goal of achieving emotional and physical integration of the patient. The work and history of Reich is developed and related to dance therapy. This paper proposes the establishment of Reich's theories and techniques as a theoretical framework for the practice of dance therapy in the Chacian modality.

Prettyman, Meryl. *Status of Dance/Movement Therapy in Brazil (Rio de Janeiro).* University of California, Los Angeles, 1994.(SP)

Prud'homme, Sarah A. *Using Dance Therapy To Address Recurrent Themes In Eating Disorders: A Study of Maria.* Antioch/New England Graduate School, 1993.

It is suggested that dance therapy is an especially appropriate modality for the eating disorder population. Recurrent themes in eating disorders are identified in a literature review and in a case study of one individual. Twenty-five dance therapy sessions with one client are grouped thematically with a description of how each theme was addressed. The author's own journal as an intern is interwoven into the discussion. It is observed that it is useful to have practical knowledge of interventions with each theme, but it is emphasized that the necessary embodiment of the mind/body connection occurs in a safe relationship with the dance therapists and the client or group members. Parallels are drawn between the thematic process of the client and the author's dance therapy internship. It is also determined that themes evolve organically in a developmental sequence without prior imposition of a particular model. The importance of the concept of connection in terms of the Stone Center relational model is considered briefly. In conclusion dance therapy is found to be an appropriate method of working with eating disorders.

Pupello, Patricia Ann. *A Dance/Movement Therapy Model of Intervention With Victims of Child Abuse*. University of California, Los Angeles. 1996.

This thesis explores the growing child's dance of life from a perspective that infants move in a world nourished by their social environment. The author hypothesizes that children who are victims of an abusive upbringing manifest certain movement characteristics that impede their ability to interact and relate optimally in society without effective healing interventions. A model of therapeutic intervention was implemented to explore the consequences of these crucial early experiences. A conceptual foundation of movement, psychotherapy and developmental theories are incorporated to build a dance/movement therapeutic framework for children traumatized by an abusive environment. During a nine month period, the four children's spontaneous dances demonstrated that current emotional and developmental consequences, psychological impairments, defensive mechanisms, and interpersonal skills can be worked through on a non-verbal, symbolic and physical level in dance/movement therapy.

Quealy, Mary Lisa. *Shamanism and Dance Therapy: Exploring the Roots of Healing*. Naropa Institute, 1996.

The premise of this thesis is that an integrated understanding of shamanism and dance therapy can yield an enriched understanding of the healing process, and can offer dance therapy an enriched perspective and enlivened therapeutic approach. This is a theoretical thesis. The intention is to look at underlying principles, theories, and paradigms of reality and healing. There is a particular interest in the potential of modern dance therapy to reclaim vital power of its original source, ancient shamanic roots.

The design of the thesis is three fold: 1) an introductory chapter for each field covering a definition, review of literature, paradigm, history, fundamental therapeutic approaches, and a summation of the healing process; 2) a discussion of the essential similarities and differences, focusing on paradigms of healing, social and historical roots, therapeutic approaches, applications, cultural contexts, and methodologies. Intentions, perspectives, techniques, working with internal and external dimensions, altered states, time and space, and consciousness are discussed; 3) the conclusion contains a summation statement, a discussion of implications, potentials, and possibilities.

Radcliffe, Nicholas. *Dance Therapy as a Primary Therapy: The Many Uses of Dance Therapy with the Dual Diagnosis Client*. Hunter College, 1985.

This paper describes a course of dance therapy with a group of developmentally disabled, emotionally disturbed adolescents, known as "dual diagnosis" clients. The particular requirements of working with the dual diagnosis client are explored, and background information about this population is included. The account draws upon theories of movement therapy and dance, and also utilizes the perspectives of theorists of teaching, social work, psychology and psychiatry. Incorporated is the view that a broad knowledge of therapy techniques will prove most effective when used in concert with a firm grasp of the particular therapy goals of the client or of the group.

Ran, Faye. *Self Esteem and Resolution of Conflicting Communication.* Hunter College, 1979.

The hypothesis of this study was that given conflicting communications through verbal and nonverbal channels, individuals with low self esteem would be more sensitive to non-verbal cues than individuals with high self esteem.

Rasmussen, Tina. *Empathy: A Comparative Study of Dance/Movement Therapy and Social Work.* Goucher College, 1994.

The purpose of this study is to identify how empathy is viewed and used by dance/movement therapists and social workers in the therapeutic process and what implications this might have for the dual degree professional (one who practices both dance/movement therapy and social work). Empathy is defined and the process of how one understands and uses empathy in the therapeutic process is explored. An introduction to both dance/movement therapy and social work with their definitions, history, principles, goals and processes are discussed. The chapters on dance/movement therapy and social work also focus on the concept of empathy as used in each of these disciplines. Five dance/movement therapists and five social workers are individually interviewed about their understanding and use of empathy in their clinical work. The results are presented in narrative form and are analyzed and discussed in terms of the similarities and differences of empathy in the therapeutic process which can be identified between dance/movement therapists and social workers. Additionally, implications of this analysis are discussed for the dual degree professional.

Ray, Diane. *Movement Characteristics of Childhood Schizophrenia.* Hunter College, 1973.

A 40 min. film on childhood schizophrenia and two shorter films on infantile autism were viewed for the purpose of recording movement and then compared through Martha Davis' diagnostic scale.

Raynor, Robyn Mae. *Dance Therapy and Children with Autism: A Theoretical Framework.* Hunter College, 1995.

Children with autism have many unique behaviors and characteristics and thus have certain needs. The purpose of this thesis is to identify and propose the field of dance therapy as a treatment modality for children with autism. This paper reviews an extensive body of literature about autism. The literature includes descriptions of behaviors, various discussions of etiological theories, as well as past and current treatment modalities. As a result of the literature review, this paper presents a theoretical framework that supports dance therapy as a treatment method which meets the special needs of children with autism.

Reed, Rosemary S. *The Dynamics of Touch and Applications with Sexually Abused Children in Dance/Movement Therapy: A Literature Review.* Allegheny University of the Health Sciences (formerly Hahnemann University), 1992.

This project involves an exploration of the significance touch has on developmental and socialization processes. The identification of touch-related disturbances are investigated. Children who have been sexually abused are at a high risk for touch-related disturbances. Treatment for these children is discussed as to when touch may serve as a therapeutic intervention in movement therapy as well as contraindications. Findings show that although touch is a primary need for all humans and may be utilized therapeutically for specific reasons, its misuse can be extremely detrimental, especially in the therapeutic context. A call for further research in the use of touch is terms of developmental stage and sex of the client and therapist is offered.

Rice, Rebecca. *The Application of Dance/Movement Therapy in Community Rehabilitation for the Chronically Mentally Ill.* Goucher College, 1994.

The purpose of this thesis is to study whether providing dance/movement therapy may be an effective therapy in psychosocial rehabilitation settings for the chronically mentally ill. The author reviews the literature on the development and practice of modern psychosocial rehabilitation, with a particular emphasis on its philosophical roots and present goals. Also reviewed is the dance/movement therapy literature to compare its definitions, histories, principles, approaches, goals, and techniques to those of the rehabilitation field. This review revealed numerous similarities in the approach of these disciplines. The author compiled and evaluated the questionnaire responses of staff and clients at several community rehabilitation centers, both with and without dance/movement therapy programs, to assess the subjects' perceptions of the benefits and drawbacks of dance/movement therapy. The author also interviewed staff and clients at these centers to obtain to identify potential obstacles that might be encountered in offering dance/movement therapy in these settings. Dance/movement therapy groups were observed at the centers offering this service to explore the possible relationship between specific dance/movement therapy techniques and specific rehabilitation goals. That dance/movement therapy can compliment rehabilitation goals and help clients obtain a more complete therapeutic and rehabilitative experience was confirmed by the results of this study. This research identified specific dance/movement therapy techniques that may be particularly useful in facilitating rehabilitation goals and noted potential obstacles that may be encountered in applying dance/movement therapy in rehabilitation settings. Dance/movement therapy was viewed by all subjects to be particularly helpful in the development of self-esteem, improving attentiveness, learning to follow directions, and in communicating and feeling connected to others. It was viewed as least helpful in the management of symptoms and in learning to make decisions. An obstacle in the application of dance/movement therapy in community rehabilitation was staff's concern of the therapeutic orientation of dance/movement therapy.

Rider, Malaya L. *The Prospective Role of Movement Therapy in Holistic Mind/Body Medicine: As Exemplified by Its Application with the Cancer Population.* University of California, Los Angeles, 1995.

This thesis explores the use of movement therapy in the growing field of holistic mind/body medicine as exemplified by its application with the cancer population. The history of biomedicine and the contributions of biology, physics, stress research and psychoneurimmunology towards a more holistic approach to health and illness are reviewed. It is proposed that the shift of attention from a strict biomedical paradigm to a synthesis of holistic and biomedical practices opens up an arena where movement therapy can grow within the medical field and be integrated.

The basic principles, goals and benefits of movement therapy are discussed and those principles that movement therapy and holistic medicine share are highlighted. Movement therapy as applied to a variety of medical conditions is discussed.

Research regarding the psychological profile of cancer patients and survivors is examined to better understand the specific needs of this population. Complementary therapies which share commonalities with movement therapy are analyzed in their application to the cancer community to support the use of movement therapy with this population.

Information obtained through questionnaires and personal interviews from movement therapists working with cancer patients is presented. A model for the use of movement therapy with the cancer population is proposed.

Rieder, Alice Suzanne. *Body and Movement Correlations to Diagnostic Criteria in the DSM-III-R.* Naropa Institute, 1994.

This thesis investigates the body and movement correlations to eight specific diagnostic categories in the DSM-III-R: disruptive behavior disorders, anxiety disorders, eating disorders, schizophrenia, mood disorders, substance abuse and personality disorders. It explores the questions: 1) Is there a body and movement correlation to these diagnostic categories? and 2) How can body and movement observations help defend or discriminate a diagnoses?

The review of literature discusses the body-based psychotherapeutic documentation of body and movement correlations to these categories, as well as assessment abilities specific to dance/movement therapy and other body-based modalities.

The documentation from the review of literature is combined with body and movement observations gathered from personal interviews with eleven dance/movement therapists and eleven traditional psychotherapists, to present how the body and movement observations do correlate to these specific diagnostic categories. The appendix includes examples of assessment forms to aid documentation of these body and movement observations.

Rikita, Cally. *Dance/Movement Therapy: A Common Vocabulary.* Columbia College, 1995.

This text is the first dance movement therapy dictionary. Included in this dictionary are definitions for terms unique to the field of dance movement therapy as well as definitions for terms that may be used by many fields but take on a specific meaning in reference to dance movement therapy. For example, a layman might think of armor as a suit of metal plates worn by knights in medieval times while a dance movement therapist would use the term armor to refer to one's total pattern of chronic muscular tension in the body. This dictionary explains these special terms. This text can be an asset to dance movement therapy students and professionals as well as any other individual interested in dance movement therapy.

Risher, Elise Ann. *Zen and the Art of Dance Therapy.* Hunter College, 1991.

This thesis examines the connection between Zen and dance therapy in order to expand the current theoretical framework of dance therapy. The literature on Zen is examined and it's major concepts are outlined including Zen's focus on the non-verbal, non-intellectual aspects of experience, its emphasis on discipline and how that discipline leads to a spontaneous, intuitive, process oriented approach to life. The literature comparing Zen and psychotherapy is examined. The literature is divided into those articles that compare theoretical concepts of Zen to psychotherapy and those articles that apply Zen concepts and techniques to the process of psychotherapy. The discussion focuses on the aspects of dance therapy that relate to Zen, namely, the concept of the unity of body and mind and the focus on a non-verbal, experiential approach that stresses spontaneity and intuition.

The field of dance therapy developed out of the combination of modern dance techniques and psychological theories. Psychology does not address those phenomenon that are unique to dance therapy such as the concept of body-mind unity, the direct physical expression of emotion and the nonverbal process of effecting change. It appears that dance therapists must looks outside psychology for a conceptual framework that addresses theseimportant aspects of the dance therapy process. The paper concludes with possible applications of Zen to dance therapy and suggests that Zen may provide another basis for a theoretical framework of dance therapy.

Rivi, Diamond. *A Study Comparing Mother-Child Dance/Movement Therapy and Individual Dance/Movement Therapy in the Treatment of Children Diagnosed with Pervasive Developmental Disorders.* Allegheny University of the Health Sciences (formerly Hahnemann University), 1996.

Dance/movement Therapy (D/MT) has been successfully applied in the treatment of children diagnosed with Pervasive Developmental Disorders (PDD) including its most severe form, autism. Traditionally, dance novement therapists have worked individually with these children and gains made in therapy were not necessarily reinforced at home. In an effort to influence children's home environment, this study devised a family-based approach which involved working with children diagnosed with PDD/autism and their mothers. It was hypothesized that including mothers in the D/MT process would lead to greater positive changes in mother-child interactions than would individual D/MT. The subjects were four children, ages three to four, and their mothers. Two children received six weekly sessions of dyadic D/MT and two children received six weekly sessions of individual D/MT. Each dyad was rated pre-and post therapy on the Non-Verbal Assessment for Family Systems (Dulicai, 1977), and each child on the Relationship to an Adult Scale from the Behavior Rating Instrument for Autistic and other Atypical Children (Ruttenberg et.al., 1977). Results at post-test showed that as a group, the children and mothers who received dyadic D/MT demonstrated greater positive change in behaviors which served the interaction and greater positive change in the quality of the mother-child interaction than did the children who received individual D/MT and their mothers. The results support the study's hypothesis. The positive results of this pilot study suggest that this design be replicated using a larger sample and follow-up assessments to explore the maintenance of treatment gains over time.

Rochell, Doran M. *Dance/Movement Therapy And Aikido: Healing And Integration With The Sexual Trauma Population.* Antioch/New England Graduate School, 1991.

This thesis proposes the use of dance/movement therapy as a healing tool to affect change in our attitudes toward the natural environment. The thesis contrasts present day attitudes toward the earth with alternative perspectives. It discusses from a feminist perspective some of the causes for this present view as well as some of the resistance that exists to change. For the survival of the natural environment, this thesis recommends that we adopt some of the alternative perspectives. Dance/movement therapy provides an opportunity for clients to grow in their understanding of their connections to their body. This thesis recommends that dance/movement therapists take this opportunity to enhance their clients' understanding of their connection not only to their bodies but to the larger cosmos.

Romer, Meryl Beth. *The Use of the Therapist's Intentional Self-Disclosure as a Tool for Eliciting the Client's Direct Experience of Self.* Naropa Institute, 1993.

This thesis explores the hypothesis that intentional and therapeutic self-disclosure on the part of the therapist serves as a tool for eliciting the client's direct experience of self. This is studied in the context of the therapeutic relationship. This author has elected to look at the various types of self-disclosure that can be utilized; and to explore the function of these methods within the framework of therapeutic relationship.

The literature review includes a study of self-disclosure, direct experience, a brief tie-in with developmental theory and research into the compatibility of this hypothesis with the substance abuse population. The methods include twenty-five session studies that look at the effects of self-disclosure within a session. This author advocates that self-disclosure, used intentionally within the framework of therelationship, has a positive and direct effect on the client's direct experience of self.

Rose, Sharon Clay. *Bridging the Generations: Intergenerational Dance/Movement Therapy.* Columbia College Chicago, 1994.

This is a case study decribing the use of dance/movement therapy in shared movement sessions. There were a series of eight sessions with five older adults in an adult day care setting. Each of the adults had some form of dementia. The five children were from a kindergarten program housed in the same day care center. The setting was an intergenerational day care center which sought to bring young children and older adults together on a daily basis. Dance/movement therapy provided a model for positive interaction between these two groups.

The thesis examines the current state of intergenerational day care, characteristics of the elderly and and young children in light of developmental theories and dance/movement therapy and its potential for each of these groups in such a setting. A description of eight sessions form the basis for a practical as well as a theoretical understanding of the contribution dance/movement therapy makes to quality intergenerational programming.

It is hoped that the information will be useful to both dance/movement therapists and to day care professionals grappling with ways to promote intergenerational care.

Rosenberg, Teddi. *A Holistic Approach to Social Group Work: A Process of Empowerment for the Severely Depressed Person.* Hunter College, 1993.

This paper explores the theories underlying the phenomenon of severe depressive disorders of the ego. It further seeks to demonstrate the value of using dance/movement therapy techniques and social group work as a catalyst for empowering the person suffering from this disease. It seeks to show the importance of a holistic approach to treating the severely depressed person which may include the use of medication and electric convulsive treatment.

Rothermel, Lynn. *Movement Integration.* California State University, Hayward, 1992.

This thesis presents an approach to psychophysical integration based on authentic expression and awareness in movement art experience. Movement as used, signifies not only the physical modality (body movement) but also the ongoing flow of subjective (inner) experience. The objective mind and subjective process are simultaneously engaged in the art experience. The observing self functions as witness to one's authentic process in order to facilitate integration of the person through integration of the objective and subjective realms of the self.

Rozen, Lynn M. *Synthesis of Theoretical Concepts in Dance/Movement Therapy and Chaos Theory.* Antioch/New England Graduate School, 1993.

Chaos Theory, a branch of Dynamical Systems Theory, is a model in mathematics that recently is being applied in psychology and movement research. Chaos Theory views elements of a system as inherently interconnected. Chaos Theory focuses on the process of a system's evolution over time rather than focusing on static state. It is a modeling strategy that allows the researcher to take multiple variables into account and to map qualitative changes in a system's state visually on a computer. The intent of the paper is to introduce Chaos Theory to the dance/movement therapy community. The paper presents basic concepts in Chaos Theory and explores philosophical parallels between Chaos Theory and theory and practice in dance/movement therapy. Suggestions for potential applications of Chaos Theory to DMT research are given. The author believes that Chaos Theory holds promise for opening new avenues for research in dance/movement therapy.

Rubenstein, Joan. *The Therapeutic Use of Movement Performance In Groups.* Hunter College, 1989.

Rumrill, Maria Rose. *Alexithymia and Dance/Movement Therapy.* Goucher College, 1993.
   This study is designed to explore the effectiveness of utilizing dance/movement therapy as a treatment modality for alexithymia. Literature in the areas of alexithymia and dance/movement therapy are reviewed. In alexithymia, definition, history, theory, and treatment are reviewed. Similarly, the dance/movement therapy literature examines definition, history, principles, goals and process. Based on the integration of this material, a theoretical case is made for the use of dance/movement therapy in treating alexithymia. Dance/movement therapy can be used in specifically addressing the areas of affect labeling, imagery and establishment of relationships in the treatment of the alexithymic patient. In order to explore this subjective material, seven chemically dependent veterans participated in six weekly one-hour dance/movement therapy sessions at an outpatient substance abuse clinic. The Toronto Alexithymia Scale (TAS) was used in a pre-test, post-test single subject design. Data analysis results revealed a decrease in alexithymic characteristics following the intervention of dance/movement therapy. Observation of sessions were made based on specific guidelines related to affect, imagery, relationship and clinical interventions. These observations were developed into a treatment overview and case vignettes which provide specific examples of the use of dance/movement therapy in treating alexithymia. The results of this study support the indications in the literature that body-oriented therapies such as dance/movement therapy are effective treatment modalities for alexithymia.

Rupp Angela. *A Case Study of an Adolescent Female Utilizing Dance/Movement Therapy as the Primary Approach.* California State University, Hayward, 1992.
   Using dance/movement therapy, the interventions facilitated expression of this adolescent's internal emotional process as well as to enable the verbal process. It was effective in addressing central issues related to anorexia nervosa. Overall, she was able to experience an increased sense of bodily integration, a greater sense of spontaneity and self assertion, and wider range of emotional expression.

Russell, Marcie. *The Use of Dance/Movement Based Support Groups to Address Occupational Stress Among Pediatric Nurses.* Allegheny University of the Health Sciences (formerly Hahnemann University), 1996.
   The hypothesis of this study is that dance/movement based support groups would decrease negative effects of stress among pediatric nurses. Nurses are under extreme stress and have immense responsibility for the well being of others. Dance/movement therapy has techniques to efficiently combat the effects of stress as well as facilitating the development of supportive relationships. Control and experimental groups were utilized and pre and post tested. Each group had 4 subjects. Five sessions were held over a period of six weeks. Each session was approximately 40 minutes and consisted of body awareness, relaxation techniques, guided imagery and improvisational and structured movement experiences. Two methods of measurement were utilized, the Lefebvre and Sandford Strain Questionnaire (SQ) (Lefebvre and Sandford, 1985) and the Feedback Form developed by this author. The experimental group's SQ score decreased by a mean of 24.5 while the control group's SQ score increased by a mean of 2.0. All responses from the Feedback Form supported the usefulness of this type of group for this population. This study supports the hypothesis that dance/movement based support group decreases the effects of stress for this population of nurses. Further study a) will need to account for the variable of race and how it relates to both social support and perception of

work place stress, and b) compare this group's effectiveness with other methods of stress relief.

Ruth, Tiffany T. *The Theoretical Application of a Developmental Model to the Theory and Practice of Dance/Movement Therapy.* Allegheny University of the Health Sciences (formerly Hahnemann University), 1994.

This study attempts to utilize the development landscape model proposed by Waddington (1957) for a theoretical investigation of developmental processes in the field of dance/movement therapy. The study begins with an investigation of the historical support for this application of bio-development (i.e. Waddingon's landscape model) to psychological development and developmental changes. Processes are studied in relation to the evolutionary thinking found in Waddington's development landscape model. The degree to which these bio-developmental processes can be and are used by dance/movement therapists is examined for implications for the theoretical base and practice of dance/movement therapy.

Samuels, Adrienne. *Dance/Movement Therapy: A Means of Expanding Social Interaction with Institutionalized Aged.* Hunter College, 1986.

Dance/movement therapy is a viable treatment for elderly individuals living in a nursing institution. Social theories of aging will provide the context in which to perceive aspects of the aging process. The results of multiple losses, institutional living and aging in general have a profound effect psychologically and on the movement repertoire of elderly people. This directly effects their ability to interact with others and in general cope in their environment. The basic premise of this paper is that dance/movement therapy can work with the psycho-social needs of the elderly and can help reconnect the individual back into some social milieu.

Sargent, Laura. *An In-Depth Exploration of Dance/Movement Therapy From A Relational Perspective.* Antioch/New England Graduate School, 1995.

The Stone Center's relational model is a therapeutic framework that emphasizes the importance of relationship, or more specifically, connection, in women's healing and growth. Central concepts defined by this model are mutual empathy, mutual empowerment, authenticity, conflict (and how it is resolved), general connection and disconnection and resilience. The physical manifestations of relational theory in dance/movement therapy are explored in this study. The study qualitatively describes one individual dance/movement therapy session in the water with a female migraine sufferer. The analysis is detailed and specific, describing the movement, words, imagery, and transitions of both the patient and the therapist. Correlations are drawn between the Kestenberg Movement Profile terms and interpretations and the above said rational concepts. The impact on the therapy of the setting (the water medium) and the patient's chronic pain issues are explored. Recommendations for further research are suggested.

Sawyer, Amanda Dobson. *"The Serendipity Circle: Inside Out" Session One of Eight. A Dance/Movement Therapy Video Pilot Series For Latency Age Children.* Antioch/New England Graduate School, 1992.

The author presents a single sample video session of a series of eight. Each video session contains six segments which are repeated in each subsequent video session but contain different content. A sample session of the pilot series is presented demonstrating implementation and utilization of dance/movement therapy to address the latency issues of Post Traumatic Stress Disorder, depressive symptomatology, and ordinary pre-adolescent pressures evidenced in latency-aged children. Enhancing an internal sense of safety and establishing confidence in ability to care in the latency age child is a key goal, hence "securitrust". The structural framework demonstrates a concrete framework based on developmental movement phases formulated by Mahler, Laban and Kestenberg, object relations, and Jungian perspectives. The author seeks to utilize movement as an activity to create self-discovery, self-esteem, personal will and securitrust within each child.

Scapini-Burrell, Isabella. *Analysis of Empathic and Countertransference Reactions of the Therapist in a Dance/Movement Therapy Session with MICA Clients.* Hunter College, 1994.

This paper investigates empathic and countertransference phenomena experienced by the beginning therapist in relation to a dance/movement therapy group of MICA (mentally ill chemically abusing) clients. The group consisted of four clients, one female and three males, who ranged between the ages of 31 and 36. 28 minutes of a videotaped dance/movement therapy session was analyzed, and countertransference reactions in movement were identified. Countertransference reactions arose in relation to 1) the client's inability to become fully involved in the movement, 2) the clients' indirect expression of rage at this therapist and 3) the client's lack of boundary awareness. It is concluded that this group needs the therapist as a mirroring self object. The leader needs to use more direct verbal observations. The beginning therapist's struggle to contain and channel the clients' hostile impulses and the importance of awareness of countertransference reactions in movement are discussed.

Scarth, Susan C. *Dance Movement Therapy with Battered Women.* Laban Centre for Movement and Dance, 1992.

Schalkwijk-Vanderkruk, Malita E. *Educational Interventions in Dance/Movement Therapy with Chronic Pain Patients.* Goucher College, 1993.

In this study, the author examines dance/movement therapists use of an educational approach within dance/movement therapy sessions when treating patients who suffer from chronic pain. The literature review provides information: 1) on pain, in particular chronic pain and its treatment within a multidisciplinary approach; 2) on psychoeducation and it's use in the treatment process of chronic pain patients; and 3) on dance/movement therapy as a profession and as a treatment modality. Finally a brief description is given on the use of dance/movement therapy as a treatment modality for chronic pain.

Ten dance/movement therapists that have worked or are currently working with chronic pain patients were interviewed by telephone utilizing a questionnaire developed by this writer. The questions were designed to elicit information on how these therapists utilize psychoeducation in their sessions. Nine of the therapists interviewed reported that they have been utilizing education as their main tool for intervention throughout the sessions when treating chronic pain patients. The ways they utilize education in their sessions is discussed in detail. A discussion follows on the findings of the project and on the process of integrating psychoeducation into the traditional practice of dance/movement therapy.

Schindler, Sammi. *Dance/Movement Therapy as a Treatment Modality for Survivors of Incest.* University of California, Los Angeles, 1994. (SP)

Schingo, Felissa. *Improving Communication in Organizations Through Movement Interventions.* Goucher College, 1994.

The purpose of this nonverbal movement study is to determine if the movement interventions of dance/movement therapy can be utilized to improve communication problems in organizations. This study incorporates both a videotape and literature to support the author's hypothesis. The literature includes a general overview of the organizational system and describes the work group as an organizational subsystem. Various problems within organizations are discussed and how they can be resolved. Types of and barriers to organizational communication are discussed, as well as specific communication issues. Communication, as a main function and potential contributor to organizational growth, is described. A section on nonverbal behavior, communication and assessment defines nonverbal communication and its relation to the organizational setting. For the purposes of this study, the author explores the nonverbal communication aspect of body movement in greater depth. The videotape consists of five vignettes which exemplify typical communication problems in organizations. Four subjects, two men and two women between the ages of 30 and 62 volunteered to role play the scenarios selected by this author. Each subject was assigned specific mock scenarios to recreate based on written information containing a general description of the subject's character. The mock scenarios were taken from the literature which described four communication issues in organizations: 1) status/power of supervisor to subordinate 2) participation and power sharing 3) mixed and contradictory messages and 4) inappropriate or unintended communication. Two scenes involved all four subjects and emphasized group interaction. Three scenes involved two subjects and emphasized couple interaction. Each scene depicted how the four communication issues were manifested nonverbally by the supervisor, subordinate/or group. The author introduced interventions into each scene by using movement to improve the communication problem. The scenes were videotaped again after the movement intervention was made utilizing the same subjects.

The result is a videotape which includes voice-overs which describe the communication problem, how it is manifested in movement, a nonverbal assessment of the problem and the movement interventions used to improve the communication problem. This study suggests that the movement interventions of dance/movement therapy can be utilized to aid effectively in improving communication problems.

Schmoelz-Schappin, Nathan. *My Personal Song Of Songs: A Creative And Spiritual Journey With Anna Sokolow.* Hunter College, 1994.

This paper reviews the history and practice of the art of dance in the West over the last two millenia. The thesis has a general focus on the use of dance as a means of healing, and its specific use to support the author's personal dance experience and its effect on his own therapeutic transformation. The author discusses his self-exploratory process while working and performing with the early modern dance pioneer Anna Sokolow on her choreographic adaption of the *Song of Songs*. Three personal aspects are explored: 1) The reconnection of the author with his therapeutic tool, his body, after an unacknowledged body trauma in the form of surgery. 2) The author's spiritual return to Judaism and how the creative process helped him to integrate his beliefs into his identity. 3) The easing of the mourning process over a partnership, and the subsequent freeing of the author's ability to love.

Scholefield, Jeannette R. *Moving Toward Role Identification with Depressed/Suicidal Adolescents in Short Term Dance/Movement Therapy.* California State University, Hayward, 1991.

The purpose of this thesis is to describe the qualitative changes which took place in a group of clinically depressed and psychiatrically hospitalized adolescents. Changes were observed during the participation of two adolescents in a three week short term dance/movement therapy program designed to enhance role identification. Observations and narrative descriptions of the initial session, the fifth, and the final session are discussed. Changes noted were bodily characteristics, individual movement behaviors and interactional movement. Changes noted were considered reflective of a move toward clearer role identification. The literature review serves as as an investigation of different treatment approaches with depressed and suicidal adolescents. The outcome of the study supports the position that dance/movement therapy promotes role identification and thereby reduces depressed behaviors.

Schultz, Robert. *Centering And The Healthy Self, An Examination of The Use of Centering For Dance/Movement Therapists.* Antioch/New England Graduate School, 1992.

Dance/movement therapists prepare themselves for and conduct their therapy sessions in a variety of ways. This paper will focus on the value for therapists of becoming centered as part of their preparation and how this impacts on the desired outcome of therapy: the healthy self. Various viewpoints on what is meant by the healthy self are presented, followed by viewpoints on centering and how centering relates to the health self. Interviews with practicing therapists are presented to offer examples of how therapists prepare for their therapy sessions and a discussion follows of how the interviews relate to centering and the healthy self. The conclusions drawn form this paper are that all therapists might give consideration to a centering process as part of their preparation for and conduct of therapy sessions.

Schwartz, Cynthia. *Short Term Dance/Movement Therapy with Hospitalized Depressed Adults.* Columbia College Chicago, 1994.

This study was designed to explore the effect of the short-term dance/movement therapy group with hospitalized depressed adults. The hypothesis is that the short-term dance/movmement therapy group can help facilitate the lessening of depressive symptoms. The writer's observations of three consecutive dance/movement therapy groups documented on a movement evaluation form and patients' self-statements were used to assess changes in depressive symptomatology. Results showed that the dance/movement therapy sessions lessened symptoms of depression such as decrease in depressed mood, brightening of affect, decreased feelings of isolation and helplessness, increased interest in social acitivity, decreased anxiety and instillation of hope. Elements and methods of short-term dance/movement therapy and realistic goal setting were also explored.

Scudder, Alice Thayer. *Dancing With The Beast: A Philosophical Embodied Approach To The Resolution of Internal Conflict, Utilizing Ki And The Principles Inherent In The Art of Karate.* Antioch/New England Graduate School, 1993.

This presentation is based on the hypothesis that, in both the traditional practice of karate-do and the use of dance and movement as a therapeutic intervention, the participant initiates actions by accessing and responding to the movement of a powerful internal energy (ki). The effective shaping and managing of this energy can lead to a positive resolution of the internal conflicts that are often at the root of emotional instability and mental illness, and prevent one from experiencing personal growth and harmony.

There is an exploration of the relationship between the underlying energy of the martial arts, in particular karate-do with reference to the art of iaido, and the energy accessed and utilized in the dance/movement therapy session. The goal is to support an affiliation between these two different approaches to personal growth and the utilization of internal energy, which in seemingly contrasting methods, seem to arrive at essentially the same position of inner balance, connection, and integration thus enhancing the ability of the individual to relate to self and others in a positive manner.

Selzman, Lisa Jennifer. *Female Adolescent Body Image: A Dance Therapy Perspective With Movement Exercises For The Young Girl.* Antioch/New England Graduate School, 1990.

An examination of female adolescent body image from a dance therapy perspective is presented. Focusing primarily on early adolescence, the investigation proposes this time period is characterized by transition and conflict, involving physiological, social and psychological experiences that influence self-perception. It is also proposed that dance therapy offers a valuable theoretical base for working to develop a healthy body image. Twenty-seven movement exercises based on the preceding research and dance therapy theory are then provided for the early adolescent female, written in accessible language, to be used for developing a realistic, positive body image and an increased sense of self-worth.

Sewickley, Judith and Fledderjohn, Heidi. *An Annotated Bibliography of Dance/Movement Therapy: 1940 -1990.* Goucher College, 1991. (See Fledderjohn)

Shaban, Heidi. *The Depths of the Edges: Creative Process Through Dance Movement & Deep Sensing as Alchemical Transformation.* Lesley College Graduate School, 1993.

This thesis is a theoretical journey based on personal experiences and thoughts of the creative process through dance movement and deep sensing. Through this process a path of alchemical transformation is found. Along this path psychological blocks are encountered and worked through , as well as transpersonal experiences leading to discoveries of ecstatic states.

Ponderings on the three aspects of the Self: the body, soul, and intellect are explored with specific focus on the harmonious and disharmonious alignment and interplay of the trio. Personal struggles regarding being an artist and performer in our society, especially those regarding the continuum between product and process are examined.

The written form of this theoretical journey attempts to pay homage to the authentic voice of the soul as it interacts with the body and intellect, and to the continuum between process and product that results in an improvisational structure.

Shahar, Tova. *The Use of Imagery, Dance Movement Techniques With Anorectics.* Antioch/New England Graduate School, 1990.

The relationship between anorexia and the use of imagery in dance/movement therapy techniques is discussed in this paper. The proposed imagery techniques include the use of active imagination through guided imagery relaxation and Authentic Movement. Other preparatory methods of intervention are utilized as well and include breathing and Progressive Relaxation. The writer used two case studies to examine the influence and effect of dance/movement interventions methods. The treatment process focused on two main topics: the anorectic's body image and the anorectic's object relations. The literature covers the topics of psychodynamic aspects of anorexia, body image, the rationale for using dance/movement therapy in treatment with anorectics in general and the rationale for using imagery dance/movement intervention techniques, including some Jungian aspects, in treatment with anorectics. The Kestenberg Effort/Shape Modality and the Self Portrait drawings were utilized as diagnostic tools.

Shaw, Bodhi. *The Potential Role of Dance Movement Therapy in the Performing Arts of Dance.* Laban Centre for Movement and Dance, 1993.

Sheble, Meggan Spence. *Dance Movement Therapy: A Tool for the Transcendence of Chronic Pain.* Lesley College Graduate School, 1992.

Researched from a body/mind/spirit perspective, this thesis draws from medical theory as well as theory on body-centered psychotherapy, the psychology of loss and transcendence, the phenomenology of pain and illness, movement therapy, death and dying, theology and suffering, and Buddhism. The physical, mental, emotional and spiritual effects of long term pain are discussed. Chronic pain is understood as an experience of loss and transcendence (overcoming loss). Dance movement therapy with art, writing and sound therapy are applied in a case study as a vehicle for the transcendence of chronic pain.

Sheppard, Paula E. *Becoming a Dance Therapist: A Case Study of Personal Growth.* Hunter College, 1984.

This paper begins with the hypothesis that personal growth is an integral and important part of training. The author surveys the literature on the training of dance therapists and group psychotherapists to find out how educators view the role of personal growth. She then reconstructs a narrative of her own experience as a student in dance therapy training group. Training was found to facilitate emotional growth by helping the student to become aware of and to resolve interpersonal difficulties that would otherwise detract from leadership effectiveness.

The specific issues that arose for the author during training were: distrust of peer group members, fear of self-disclosure, need for group acceptance, vulnerability toward and over-dependence on the group, and transference toward instructors. The two activities that were found to be most helpful for resolving these difficulties were introspective log-keeping and process commentary discussions. The growth process that took place during training was found to provide the author with a new level of interpersonal ease—one that positively influenced not only her professional interactions, but also her personal relationships.

Sherrill, Jonna M. *Defense Mechanisms and Muscular Tension: A Dance/Movement Therapy Perspective and Survey of Health Professionals.* Naropa Institute, 1993.

The present investigation examines the signs of psychological defense mechanisms in an individual and questions if professionals in the fields of medicine and psychology have observed the presence of skeletal muscle tension in situations which may call for defensive reactions. The intention is to show the relationship between psychological defense mechanisms and skeletal muscle tension. The ideas of somatic theorists and dance/movement therapists are presented here for support of this proposed relationship.

The author has created and distributed a questionnaire/survey on this hypothesis to various professionals in the fields of health and psychology. Upon analysis of 15 completed and returned questionnaires, these professionals have reported observing defense mechanisms as well as various kinds of muscular tension. Also reported was a positive correlation between these two factors as observed in clients. From the ideas of other theorists and results of the completed survey, a positive correlation has been shown to exist between defense mechanisms and tension in skeletal muscle.

Simon, Jennifer. *Dance Therapy and the Deaf Population.* Hunter College, 1996.

This paper focuses on how to use dance therapy as a hearing therapist working with a deaf adult psychiatric population. The term deaf in this paper refers to individuals who have any impairment in hearing words and sounds. The paper is divided into sections discussing dance therapy, the deaf community, methods of communication, the psychology of deafness, history of deaf mental health services, types of diagnosis, the therapeutic relationship, transference and counter-transference, use of dance with the deaf, and use of dance therapy with the deaf. Based on this author's experience, the deaf population can benefit a great deal from dance therapy.

Simpson, Amanda. *An Exploration of Dance Movement Therapy with a Group of Borderline Personality Disorder Clients.* Laban Centre London, 1996.

This thesis considers the role dance movement therapy may play with borderline personality clients. The methodological approach used for this thesis is a qualitative one, synthesizing aspects of heuristic and phenomenological research methods. The study consists of a series of clinical descriptions of dance movement therapy work with a small group of six clients holding the diagnosis of borderline personality disorder, placed in a hospital day unit. Three themes are discussed: 1) The 'holding environment' and its potential healing role in dance movement therapy with the borderline personality client. 2) The significance of the cyclical theme of advance and retreat and what it may be both serving and symbolizing for the borderline personality disorder client. 3) Finding the middle ground of the 'True Self' (Winnicott 1965) and how to facilitate the experience of the 'True Self' in the borderline client, which lies between the defensive extremes of either impulsive catharsis or listless passivity. The thesis concludes by describing the implications this information may have on approaches and techniques that might usefully be integrated in future dance movement therapy work with this population.

Smith, Pamela. *Three Case Studies on the Use of Dance Therapy with Autism and Pervasive Development Disorders Including Neurological Implications of Autistic Syndromes.* Hunter College, 1995.

This thesis incorporates three individual case studies on children diagnosed with Pervasive Developmental Disorders and Autistic features. Dance/movement therapy is used as a therapeutic intervention for working with each child. The neurological aspects of their developmental disorders are considered in how dance therapy may help improve their learning capabilities and organization of the world. Individual progress is assessed through session logs, progress reports, and individual testing. Neurological functioning theories are adapted in an attempt to discuss possible causes for developmental difficulties and possible interventions for improving development using dance therapy. It was found that individual dance therapy sessions did help improve social interactions and relations to people, organization of thoughts and sensory input, improved eye contact and focus on activities, and increased body and spatial awareness. Learning improved within individual dance therapy sessions, and all three children progressed in relation to dance therapy interventions used.

Steckert, Kimberly. *Case Study of an Attention-Deficit/Hyperactive Child Exhibiting Poor Body Boundaries.* University of California, Los Angeles, 1996. (SP)

Steinberg, Sheila. *Dance Therapy with a Chronic Paranoid Schizophrenic from a Developmental View: A Case Study.* New York University, 1985.

In this case study of a 55 year old chronic paranoid schizophrenic woman with somatic complaints, the benefits of working with a developmental dance therapy approach are described. Schizophrenia, psychosis, hallucination and delusion are defined, with an emphasis on the latter. The oral phase, fixation point of schizophrenia is discussed. Target behaviors are described for each of the seven dance therapy sessions held with the patient, charted and graphed in terms of strength and deficits. Overall results show a positive growth in strength from baseline observations. The single case experimental design is suggested for more vigorous testing of developmental dance therapy techniques with the schizophrenic patient.

Steinberger, Debja. *Cultivating Joy in the Early Stages of Recovery From Addiction Using Dance/Movement Therapy.* Antioch/New England Graduate School, 1991.

This paper describes the transformative power of joy in reclaiming one's life from the bondage of addiction. Shame and guilt are invasive emotions which appear to entrap the addict in a self defeating world. These toxic emotions are viewed as the shadow side of joy, destroying any functions of health, vitality, and the authentic self. The dance/movement therapy session is revised discussing the facilitation of surrender as a necessary and important part of recovery to claiming joy, a creative life, and long term sobriety. A central focus is the use of dance/movement therapy in conjunction with the twelve steps.

Stent, Denise. *Dance/Movement Therapy and Childhood Autism.* University of California, Los Angeles, 1994.(SP)

Stepek, Heather Lee. *Dance/Movement Therapy: A Profile of the Field.* Allegheny University of the Health Sciences (formerly Hahnemann University), 1995.

The objective of this study is to derive an Occupational Personality Profile of dance/movement therapists who have obtained the ADTR (Academy of Dance Therapists Registered) level of registry. Using the Occupational Personality Questionnaire (Saville & Holdsworth Ltd., 1984-1987) and a brief supplemental demographic survey, ADTR's attending the 1994 national conference of the ADTA were surveyed. Due to a low number of responses, additional subjects were recruited from the Pennsylvania and nearby chapters of the ADTA for a total of 34 respondents. Results showed that the dance/movement therapists surveyed scored high on the independent, caring, artistic, behavioral, conceptual, and worrying scales. They indicated low scores on the persuasive, controlling, data rational, forward planning, detail conscious, conscientious, relaxed, tough-minded, emotional control, competitive, achieving, and social desirability scales. These findings indicate that although well matched for the service aspect of the profession, the occupational personality of dance/movement therapists as a group shows limitations of the field and its potential for growth in the marketplace. This data will be useful when seeking ways to motivate individuals within the field to respond to government alerts and to increase publication. It also provides graduate schools with more discerning criteria to look for in prospective students in order to select new members who will be strong contributors to the field of dance/movement therapy.

Stern, Hillary. *Treating Eating Disorders: A Focus on the Body.* Hunter College, 1996.

Stone, Robyne. *Dancing to Your Own Rhythm: A Step-By-Step Guide for Developing a Private Practice in Dance/Movement Therapy.* Goucher College, 1993.

The purpose of this study is to establish a guide for dance/movement therapists to develop a private practice. A background review of the literature written on the current trend of mental health professionals who are leaving agency settings and entering private practice is provided. The primary business aspects of setting up a private practice are discussed, and the challenges specific to dance/movement therapists establishing a private practice are compared to those facing other mental health professionals.

A questionnaire was created which was mailed to thirty dance/movement therapists throughout the country. The questionnaire consisted of questions relevant to the individual experiences of dance/movement therapists as they established themselves in private practice. Ten questionnaires were returned, but only eight were applicable to the study. These eight questionnaires, in addition to literature on private practice written by other mental health professionals, were combined to form the foundation for a 15 step guide for developing a private practice in dance/movement therapy. The guide is able to offer several suggestions to obstacles faced by dance/movement therapists in private practice. The small sample size makes it difficult to generalize the results of the study.

Stone, Sheila McDevitt. *Dance/Movement Therapy with Families: A Comparison of Psychoanalytic and Humanistic Family Therapy.* Allegheny University of the Health Sciences (formerly Hahnemann University), 1995.

The practice of family therapy is diverse, consisting of numerous distinct paradigms. Dance/movement therapy with families does not base its work on a particular paradigm, but is eclectic in nature. This thesis explores the similarities of dance/movement therapy with families with two specific family therapy paradigms—psychoanalytic and humanistic family therapy. The psychoanalytic family therapy theory and practice presented is based on the work of Nathan Ackerman. The work of Virginia Satir is the basis for the exploration of humanistic family therapy theory and practice. The work of these particular therapists/theorists are compared to dance/movement therapy, as well as research and the practice of dance/movement therapy with families. This thesis validates and justifies the practice of dance/movement therapy with families by clearly delineating theoretical underpinnings from psychoanalytic and humanistic family therapy. The literature explored in this thesis demonstrates similarities in theoretical and practical frameworks of both Ackerman and Satir in relation to the theory and practice of dance/movement therapy with families.

Strickler, Sari Allyn. *The Neutral Zone: A Theoretical Paradigm Dance/Movement Therapy for Hearing Parents and Deaf Children.* Hunter College, 1995.

This thesis explores DMT as an effective therapeutic modality for enhancing communication of the deaf member family system. The review of literature focuses on: the etiology and psychological development of deafness; the psychological impact on hearing parents and their deaf child; theories related to DMT and object relations; and the use of DMT with deaf children and their family system.

Integrating the theoretical frameworks of Winnicott, Satir, and Luterman with dance/movement therapy theory allows the development of a paradigm for working with this population. This preliminary study validates the use of dance/movement therapy for hearing parents and deaf children because of the use of the "neutral" language of dance.

Stupka-Malloy, Amy. *The KMP Explored: An Illustrated Presentation of The Tension-Flow Rhythms.* Antioch/New England Graduate School, 1992.

A comprehensive examination and description of the Tension-flow rhythms (a portion of the Kestenberg Movement Profile) is presented. Photographs, illustrations, and verbal descriptions are utilized. The Kestenberg Movement Profile, it is suggested, serves as a link between traditional developmental psychology and the emerging field of expressive arts therapy, providing a traditionally-based framework for the dance/movement therapist.

Sussman, Shari. *A Theoretical Approach to Unresolved Childhood Grief in Dual Diagnosed Patients and How Dance Therapy Breaks Through the Resistance to Heal.* Hunter College, 1993.

This thesis presents a theoretical approach for understanding unresolved childhood grief in dually diagnosed patients and how dance therapy breaks through the resistance to heal.Children's conception of death at various developmental stages is explored to determine consequences of unresolved grief from the death of a parent. The questions which arise include: are the psychological effects of parent loss pathological and does unresolved mourning relate to pathology? The population studied are dually diagnosed patients which includes substance abusers with a second diagnosis of depression and/or anxiety and early loss. These patients did not receive any form of therapy prior to adulthood and who chose substances to cope with grief. The existence of resistance through the body is evidence of the unconscious conflict to heal. The specific manifestations of bodily resistance are studied. Dance therapy is suggested as the optimum tool for healing this group of patients with early loss.

Sutton-Randolph, Charlese. *How Does Various Music (Gospel, Reggae, Jazz, Rock and Roll, Rhythm and Blues) Affect the African-American Clients' View of Dance Therapy?* Hunter College, 1992.

The question of music posed in this thesis was researched through reviewing African-American music and dance history, and interviewing individuals on their particular responses to dance and music programs. Thirty individuals of various ethnic backgrounds residing in a nursing home were asked their views on the effects of music in a dance therapy program. The format chosen was an informal personal interview where the individual responded with open-ended answers. The interviews were held where the individual was most comfortable, provided an atmosphere of confidentiality and respect between interviewer and interviewees. The results were then tabulated and compared to distinguish responses in terms of age, race, sex, religion, and educational backgrounds. The conclusion of this research coincides with the literature review in that the responses of African-Americans in dance therapy programs relates to a history of interaction between music and dance with the culture. Individuals of this particular ethnicity then, will respond quite naturally to music of their culture when used in a dance therapy group.

Szuszan, Marta. *Inner Fire as a Catalyst of Self Transformation.* Lesley College Graduate School, 1993.

Experiences of self-transformation have basic, essential similarities regardless of historical period or cultural background. This paper attempts to describe processes of self transformation using the "Inner Fire" metaphor in its universal meaning as reflected in the author's world, the world of flamenco. Flamenco is a whole complex of experiences: they are described mainly concentrating on the purification of body and soul as well as on the religious experience.

The author deals with the notion of fire and its relation to the idea of psychological, mental or conscious "fire." The essence and value of the experience of unity generated by and based on the inner fire is discussed. The author attempts to describe the general aspects of "fire," and more specifically, the experience of enlightenment as an aspect transpiring from the process of self transformation. The experience can be consciously and deliberately sought for and generated via the dance and the Cante Jondo.

Tangstad, Ann-Brit. *Patient Assessments and the Interface Between Physiotherapy and Dance Therapy.* Laban Centre for Movement and Dance, 1992.

Thelen, Judith A. *The Use of the Circle Formation to Facilitate the Individuation Process in Dance Therapy with an Acute Schizophrenic Population in a Short-Term Psychiatric Setting.* New York University, 1982. (C-Vol.I)

Thomas, Deborah. *The Absent Feminine and Pathological Emptiness.* Pacifica Graduate Institute, 1997. (Doctoral).
 This is a theoretical exploration of the experience of emptiness in pathology, in spiritual practice, and in the lost sacred feminine. Literature dealing with Borderline Personality Disorder, whose symptoms include feelings of emptiness, abandonment, and unbearable loneliness, was examined. Relevant literature indicated that this condition is often associated with childhood sexual abuse and that survivors are more often female. The acceptance and subsequent denial of these histories by S. Freud was described. Pathological experiences of childhood were compared with D.W. Winnicott's theory of adequate mothering. Speculations on the role of emptiness in psychotherapeutic technique were offered in an attempt to determine what is missing in a society where such abuses and pathologies occur.
 A study of the nature and role of emptiness in Buddhist meditative practices and concepts was undertaken. Two uses of emptinesss were discovered to be of significance for the practice of psychotherapy—ascetic techniques and tantric meditation. A feminist source on Buddhism revealed both an honoring of Buddhist feminine deities and misogyny in Buddhist societies. The feminine body was sometimes reviled and sometimes honored.
 The presence and absence of the sacred feminine in Judaic and Christian theological history was examined. A background feminine deity was seen to have been denied and her generative characteristics incorporated into male deities. Fundamental myths of patriarchal society were analyzed and found to involve the splitting of the female/male, body/mind, body/soul, along with subjugation and exploitation of women and the exaltation of warlike heroism.
 A feminist counter-attack on patriarchy stated that a healthy society would value the feminine, the body and the creative expression of emotions. A review of D.W. Winnicott's theories connected these elements with the infantile experience of adequate mothering. In conclusion, dance/movement therapy was described and identified as a valid psychotherapeutic approach to pathological loss of childhood, the body/soul, and thesacred feminine.

Thomas, Kaisha A. *The Healing Effects of Carnival in Trinidad and Its Relevance to Dance Therapy.* Hunter College, 1991.
 This thesis examines the history and healing effects of ritual dance and the events that led up to the Trinidad Carnival in particular. Parallels are drawn between dance therapy and Carnival, as it was evident that Carnival had positive effects on both individual people and the country as a whole. The theory behind this thesis is based on the fact that for the past one hundred and fifty years, the people of Trinidad and Tobago have been engaging in what has, within the past twenty years, been called "Dance Therapy."

Thorpe, Lee Bernstein. *Moving The Mind's Eye: Guidelines For Using Imagery In Conjunction With Dance/Movement Therapy.* Columbia College, 1992.
 A random sample survey was sent to 55 ADTR's living in the USA for the purpose of finding out in what way, if any, ADTR's used imagery, and to investigate their awareness of how they used

imagery within a dance/movement therapy session. To substantiate the foundation for the connection between dance/movement therapy and imagery, the work of three health professionals were reviewed. These were Alma Hawkins, dance/movement therapist, Bernie S. Siegel, M.D., and Emmett E. Miller, M.D., actor, poet and hypnotist. Imagery is defined and divided into the four categories of concrete images, abstract images, movement images, and personal images.

There were 22 responses out of the 55 questionnaires. 21 out of 22 found that the use of imagery in a dance/movement therapy session can substantially add to the dance/movement therapist's ability to reach the client. There are seven themes in total; two will be used as examples. 1) Psychotic individuals: concrete and movement images seem to be the best for facilitating reality based communication or not perpetuating delusions or hallucinations. 2) Individual therapy: Personal images are the most beneficial. Through imagery, the self-healing process can be stimulated by enabling the individual to use his/her imagination, which is a key factor in the creative process of healing.

Thurston, Christina J. *Treating Survivors of Trauma With Dance/Movement Therapy Using Dr.David Johnson's Developmental Model.* Antioch/New England Graduate School, 1993.

In this thesis the uses of dance/movement therapy (DMT) with trauma survivors according to Dr.David Johnson's developmental model (presented at the National Coalition of Arts Therapies Association Conference [NCATA] in November 1990) is explored. An updated definition of some symptoms of Post Traumatic Stress Disorder (PSTD) is presented using published findings from specialists in the field of psychological trauma. The information about trauma with DMT as a source of treatment according to Johnson's model is synthesized using this writer's theoretical considerations. It is this writer's opinion that it is important for a survivor to integrate their trauma, and to have hope, meaning and purpose of life. DMT is presented as a mode of treatment for survivors.

Tobler, Anna Christine. *Dance/Movement Therapy as Compared to Verbal Psychotherapy in the Treatment of Vietnam Veterans with Post-Traumatic Stress Disorder.* Goucher College, 1994.

The purpose of this study is to examine the role of dance/movement therapy in the treatment of Vietnam veterans who have been diagnosed with post-traumatic stress disorder as compared to existing forms of verbal psychotherapy treatment. The review of literature includes a discussion of post-traumatic stress disorder with respect to its presentation in Vietnam war veterans. The circumstances of the Vietnam war and the combat experience of the soldiers are covered, together with the etiology of the disorder,government sponsored approaches to treatment, and existing forms of verbal psychotherapy treatment. There is a review of dance/movement therapy, with regard to its definition, history, principles, goals, and process. There is an integration chapter exploring dance/movement therapy as it has been applied to survivors of trauma, and specifically with Vietnam veterans with post-traumtic stress disorder.

The methodology of this study was to interview both dance/movement therapists and verbal psychotherapists about their clinical work. Verbal psychotherapists were included because of the limited number of dance/movement therapists to be found who have experience in working with this population. The responses of both subject groups have been evaluated according to the similarities and differences with respect to the topics of the interview questions. All therapists responded similarly regarding their basic approach to treatment for this population, indicating that only the accompanying symptoms of PTSD can be addressed in a short term setting, with the more in depth work needing the format of a long term setting. The main differences between the two groups were in the areas of conceptualization of issues and treatment goals, and methods and techniques. This study used a very small sample size, however, it did provide valuable information which allowed the two approaches to be compared and contrasted. This study supported the hypothesis that dance/movement therapy can have a useful role in the treatment of Vietnam veterans in both short term and long term settings.

Torp, Carin. *Coming Home: Dance/Movement Therapy As a Tool For Healing Homeless Women And The Earth.* Antioch/New England Graduate School. 1994.

This thesis is based on the notion that humans are part of-rather than separate from-the whole planet Earth. Lovelock's Gaia Hypothesis, Ecofeminism and other philosophical and scientific traditions are drawn upon to support this. The assumption is made that the Earth is currently in crisis in part because the human community has lost its sense of connection to the Earth. Homeless women are the particular focus as they embody the plight we are all in- how "out of home" we are. An eight week dance movement therapy group with homeless women is set forth which draws its theoretical support from the Relational Model, Ecopsychology and Family Systems Theory. The whole thesis stresses that healing of individuals will help to heal the Earth.

Trachtenberg, Karin Grace. *Bridging the Gap: Dance Therapy in the Nursing Home.* Lesley College Graduate School, 1992.

This thesis focuses on the role of dance/movement therapy and other creative modalities within the nursing home as effective tools allowing for communication, expression and socialization. It identifies some of the issues challenging the institutionalized elderly, especially the older woman, and how the author as the dance therapist, designed activities to meet their needs. This paper is accompanied by a video tape of a special project implemented in the nursing home which explores the use of reminiscence, dance, and music to create a positive group experience; one which reinforces identity, builds self-esteem, encourages meaningful interpersonal relationships and fosters a sense of belonging. This paper describes some of the author's experiences working with the elderly and the feelings that surfaced within her as a result.

Trainor, Meg. *Dance Therapy as a Treatment Modality for Emotionally Disturbed Children within a Public School Day Treatment Setting.* Naropa Institute, 1991.

The hope is that this material may help in the clarification and informational process of day treatment programs within the public school system by focusing on special education classrooms specifically designed for emotionally disturbed children and how dance therapy can provide an integral form of treatment within this milieu.

In the two case studies presented, one is viewed from a long term perspective focusing upon our cumulative work over a nine month period of time and the other case study focuses upon the dynamics of an individual dance therapy session. These two case studies are presented to emphasize the role dance therapy can play in the integration of the child's psycho/physical development. An improved sense of body image, self awareness, self esteem, impulse control and sense of autonomy are a few of the potential benefits resultant from the dance therapy experience.

The recommendation is that dance therapy be integrated as a daily component of the treatment plan for an emotionally disturbed child. Individual dance therapy sessions are recommended as well as a regular group dance therapy experience and a rest/relaxation period. Specific diagnostic and therapeutic dance therapy exercises are presented that could be used with emotionally disturbed children in a day treatment setting. Day treatment programs within the public school systems should take advantage of a dance therapist's training and skills by incorporating them as part of the treatment team. It is to the advantage of society to implement day treatment programs within the existing structure of the public school systems and it is also advantageous to a day treatment program to integrate the skills and perspective of a dance therapist as a part of a treatment team.

Trinkley, Marcia L. *Self-in-Relation to One's Soul And The Universe: Women at Mid-Life.* Antioch/New England Graduate School, 1992.

A new approach to psychotherapy is introduced which integrates the use of feminist theory, expressive arts and the group as vessel toward the discovery of self-in-relation to one's soul and the universe. A group of four women met for the purpose of exploring their authentic selves at mid-life. Shedding the patriarchally based view of development and focusing on a new way of exploring who we are resulted in a journey of discovery. This discovery revealed the spiritual connection to one another, to nature and to the universe. Each subject made two masks, one of her inner self and one of her outer persona. The masks were viewed as representing the dichotomy between the soul connection and the patriachally based woman-in-society. Recommendations are made to use this new approach with psychotherapy/support groups of both a verbal nature and expressive arts focus.

Trott, Marjory. *Dance Therapy as a Way to Increase Self-Esteem in Adolescent Girls.* Hunter College, 1995.

The literature on adolescents, adolescent girls, cultural expectations of girls and women in America, body image, self-esteem and the problems created when it is lacking are all reviewed. Theories on how to work with adolescent girls are presented along with theliterature on dance therapy, both generally and as it relates to adolescents and the specific issues that they face. A model for using dance therapy to increase self-esteem in girls entering adolescence is developed.

Tsunemine, Yasuyo. *Overlapping Approaches of Play and Dance/Movement Therapies for a Severely, Parentally Neglected Child in a Therapeutic-Educational Setting.* University of California, Los Angeles, 1994.

This thesis attempts to document the effectiveness of play and dance/movement therapies in a therapeutic educational setting, based upon a case study carried out during an eight month internship at a Residential Therapeutic School. A discussion of the following issues provides the basis for analyzing this case: 1) the parentally neglected child (definition, etiology, effects, and general intervention), 2) treatment for parentally neglected children through play and creative arts (art, music, and dance/movement) therapies, 3) therapy and treatment goals in play and dance/movement therapies for neglected children, and 4) the counter-transference reactions by therapists working with children who are victims of severe parental neglect. This case study is based upon the author's work with a severely, parentally neglected child, re-named "Susie." Susie received treatment that combined play and dance/movement therapies. These recorded observations of the sessions and observation of Susie outside of her therapeutic sessions form the primary source material for analysis. Emphasis is placed on Susie's creative potential and her progress is chronicled. This child's emotional and behavioral responses to sessions in which play and dance/movement therapies were employed are described, as well counter-transference reactions of the author.

Tupa, Ruthann. *Ballroom Dance As Therapy From An Interpersonal/Cognitive Perspective.* Antioch/New England Graduate School, 1993.

In this thesis, ballroom dance as a dance/movement therapy modality from a cognitive perspective explores four premises: that we are continually in relationship; that through relationship we come to sense ourselves; that moving in relationship, as in dance, brings a specific awareness of ourselves and our feelings; and that recognizing and understanding these feelings is the first step toward change. The basis for these premises is found in both literature pertaining to movement and in personal observation. The conclusion drawn is that the possibility for change grows from the realization and awareness of self moving in relationship as that movement interaction fosters self knowledge of the origins of relational patterns. The cognitive theory of H.S. Sullivan, which holds that we respond to life events out of a sense of anxiety and desire for acceptance by another supports the premise that our self knowledge arises out of interpersonal interactions.

Turkenitz, Tamar. *Stages of Social Participation as it is Manifested in a Dance Therapy Session.* Hunter College, 1991.

This study explores developmental stages of social participation (interaction) as patterns of behavior that are evident in a dance therapy session with psychiatric inpatients. Stages of social participation are defined as solitary, parallel, and cooperative. A taped dance therapy session was analyzed for the presence of these social participation characteristics. The data reflects the relationship of social developmental stages within the group process of a dance therapy session. Dance therapy was found to elicit cooperative stages of social participation. The structure and the progression of the group allows each participant to experience all of the stages of social participation. Individual characteristics emerged from the consistencies of those patterns across time throughout the session.

Turner, Tracey N. *Dance/Movement Therapy in Conjunction With Storytelling as a Healing Modality For Female Perpetrators.* Antioch/New England Graduate School, 1990.

This thesis is based on limited published and unpublished material on female perpetration to expand this knowledge through the application of dance/movement therapy in conjunction with storytelling. This thesis reviews a comprehensive study of female perpetrators done by Mathews, Matthews, Speltz (1989) and a unpublished dissertation by Turner (1990). The scarcity of literature has led to a narrow theoretical focus combining the studies of sexual abuse as treated by dance/movement therapy and storytelling with the limited studies of female perpetrators.

Female perpetrators report isolation coupled with dependency on male partners. Some are pressured and coerced into abuse. Current treatment frameworks for female sexual abuse victims recognize many of the symptoms of identifying with the aggressor. In this thesis it is assumed that female perpetrators are also sexual abuse victims.

It appears that dance/movement therapy in conjunction with storytelling coud developa more effective and comprehensive approach to treatment. A model of treatment using both is presented.

Umiguchi, Yuki. *An Exploration of the Approaches of Dance Movement Therapy and Shiatsu to Muscular Tension Related to Emotional Conflicts.* Laban Centre for Movement and Dance, 1995.

Vella, Graceann E. *Case Study of a Depressed Adolescent with Borderline Syndrome in Dance/Movement Therapy.* Hunter College, 1992.

This paper's aim is to integrate the theoretical and empirical aspects of developmental theory and theories on borderline and depressive syndromes with dance therapy. An overview of an empirical and theoretical literature on depression in children and adolescents is presented. This is followed by a case study involving a depressed borderline boy, and a treatment plan implementing dance therapy treatment as an intervention for these problems. Also included are issues relevant to diagnosis and assessment. This paper suggests that there is an unequivocal relationship between depression and dance therapy as a treatment modality for individuals and groups of patients with borderline and depressive diagnoses.

Venable, Emily I. *Dance/Movement With An Adolescent Mother: A Case Study.* Allegheny University of the Health Sciences (formerly Hahnemann University), 1994.

Adolescent mothers and their infants have been identified as a high risk population. Due to the resulting economical and psychological trauma faced by the adolescent mother, she is emotionally unavailable for her infant. This case study was designed to explore and describe the process and possible benefits of dance/movement therapy with an adolescent mother in three therapeutic contexts: individual therapy, peer group therapy, and mother/infant group therapy. The sessions ran for twelve weeks with each type of therapy session meeting once a week. Clinical material was collected after each session focusing on the subject's use of touch, visual behaviors, vocalizations, proximity, mirroring, empathy and use of efforts. The adolescent answered questions regarding her feelings and impressions of the three therapeutic sessions which were compared to this clinician's findings. The hypothesis that the individual sessions and the peer group sessions would promote positive interactions between the mother and her infant was not necessarily established. However, it is within the scope of this study to note that the individual sessions appear to be the most beneficial therapeutic intervention and that the three therapeutic contexts provided the subject alternative environments in which to address her varying needs.

Vincent, Nancy Birkett. *Bridging The Gap: Quantum Leaps in Dance/Movement Therapy.* Antioch/New England Graduate School, 1992.

The main issue explored in this paper is the necessity of broadening our definition as dance/movement therapists. Against a backdrop of quantum physics, along with a more holistic medical model, dance/movement therapy is seen as one very important part of a multi-modal approach to psychotherapy. Research suggests the necessity of talking about experiences as well as embodying them to avoid isolation from oneself. By the same token, movement only, without a conscious understanding of the movement, is also limiting. Using storytelling and myth in conjunction with movement, one can not only verbalize and move with experiences and stories, but through the use of myths, access the eternal aspects of Self. Thus, one is able to work with the mind, body and spirit.

Visconti, Donna Marie. *A Case of an Emotionally Disturbed Girl.* Hunter College, 1991.

This paper presents a case study of Lara, an emotionally disturbed 7 year old Soviet Jewish girl, and includes the analysis of three videotaped dance/movement therapy sessions. When first seen, Lara was sitting amongst a room full of children, withdrawn into her coat and would haphazardly strike out with sudden vocal bursts and kicking. Lara appeared to be the most disturbed child in the room and yet she emitted the loudest non-verbal message of wanting to be heard. My goals in dance/movement therapy for Lara were to establish a trusting relationship, increase her sense of self-esteem, and enable her to acknowledge and explore her own emotions.

The literature review covers pertinent aspects of Soviet culture, theories of child development, and the use of dance/movement therapy with the abused and emotionally disturbed child. Through the use of dance/movement therapy, Lara was able to make advancements and experience trust and nurturance that she had not yet been able to fully experience with her mother and other caretakers. At the time of our last session together, Lara was beginning to verbally express the feelings she had buried deep inside.

Vorspan, Roberta. *On the Borderline.* Hunter College, 1982.

This paper is about being on the borderline of several of life's arenas. It's about the author's experience of being on the borderline between patient and therapist, dependent and independent, employed and unemployed, working through her own borderline pathology and still being in the thick of it, and finally between fighting to survive and giving up in hopelessness and defeat. The first part of the paper is a subjective account. The second part is present reflections on those experiences, theory related to borderline pathology, the therapist's use of his/her inner life in work with patients and attempts to probe the usefulness and liabilities of conflicts in work as a dance therapist.

Wallace, Jilba. *A Description of Self-Actualizing Factors in Dance/Theater Performance with Possible Implications for Dance/Movement Therapy.*
Naropa Institute, 1992.

This study investigates the experiences of two dance/theater performance groups, one with performers from a disabled population, and the other a group of higher functioning performers. Inquiries are made about six factors considered to be present in the performance process, to find out whether these performers consider them important, to what degree, and whether comparisons can be made of the experience of these factors between individuals and the two groups.

Further investigation is made to find if these factors (catharsis, self confidence, learning about oneself, receiving audience response, a sense of community and the practice of discipline towards a goal) can lead to self actualization in the performers' lives. The definitions include explanations of the performance process, the concept of self-actualization, the nature of the therapeutic contract and improvisation.

A questionnaire/interview with the core members of each group was conducted, as well as extensive interviews with the relatives and counsellors of the disabled performers. A written questionnaire related to movement behavior (the dance/movement therapy assessment) was filled out by the director of this group.

The results show similarities and differences between the individuals and the two groups, how they experienced the factors both in the performance process and in life. Conclusions indicate the value of dance/movement performance as a potential tool for self actualization, and that it can be especially applicable in the field of dance/movement therapy.

Ward, Cheryl D. *Group Dream-Work: Dancing The Dream-A Pilot Study.*
Hunter College, 1991.

This study combines group dream work and dance in order to unearth the unconscious meaning of the dream. The literature on the nature and theory of dreams as presented by Freud and Jung is reviewed. Group dream work designs of Moreno, Peris, Ullman, Shuttleworth et al., and Zinker are considered briefly focusing on each design's inherent strengths and weaknesses. The literature of Whitehouse and Chodorow identifying dance/movement as a form of Jung's "active imagination," and Mindell's "dreambody process" is reviewed.

A new five step group dream work design is created based upon the above group designs and the techniques of dance/movement therapy. This new group dream work model appears to accomplish the following:(l) provides an inroad to the dreamer's unconscious processes, (2) gathers more information and insight into felt responses, roles, and interactions for both the dreamer and group members, and (3) provides a corrective-emotional experience.

A pilot study based upon this new dream-work design was undertaken using a group comprised of one leader and five female volunteers. The eight sessions are videotaped and later reviewed. Four of the eight sessions are chosen for their ability to illustrate this new dream-work design and are discussed. Recommendations for future reproductions of this method of working with the dream within a group context are described.

Watkins, Ann R. *An Application of The Kestenberg Movement Profile and Ritual: A Case Study.* Antioch/New England Graduate School, 1995.

Throughout our lives we go through periods of personal and relational development. This thesis focuses on ten months of this phenomenon in the life of one girl in her twelfth to thirteenth year. It looks through the lens of dance/movement therapy (DMT) as experienced through the enactment of a rite of passage, bringing into consideration the "tasks of adolescence" and Relational Theory. The adolescent's emotional shifts, expressed through movement, personal presentation, and self-expression are examined using the Kestenberg Movement Profile (KMP), a tool of DMT. Turning points in her therapy are resourced from the therapist's audio-tapes, video tapes, and notes. The interventions used to facilitate those turning points are discussed.

Watney, Lucy. *A Case Study of the Effects of Dance Movement Therapy on a Child with Downs Syndrome.* Laban Centre for Movement and Dance, 1992.

Watson IV, Larkin D. *Soul Journey Discovery: Projective Identification, Brain Process and Expressive Arts Healing Dependency.* Lesley College Graduage School, 1992.

Addiction has become a culture wide epidemic now known as "dependency". This thesis presents an analysis of the dependency problem and a theory for therapy based in three levels of abstraction: the spiritual referent of soul and soul journey, the psychological referent of projective identification, and the neuro-physiological referent of brain processes, particularly in those distinctions of the bicameral neocortex, the limbic system and the proto-reptilian brain. Given these perspectives, the thesis explains why therapy of people with dependencies (and other forms of mental illness) should involve the expressive arts. Expressive arts therapy enable the dependent to re-vision his self and world images from his soul's point of view, and to re-vision his past, present and future as a soul journey. This permits the dependent person to contain the brain's multiple versions of "reality," in particular the two paradoxical versions of the neocortex, the left-brain's logical time-space "reality" and right-brains's imaginal relational-space "reality" Soul journey discovery empowers the dependent to be a "co-creator" of reality.

Two video taped examples of therapy sessions are included which highlight two apects of expressive arts therapy work on soul journey discovery: 1) the synersitic effects of multi-modal expressive arts therapy, and 2) the process of re-owning projective identifications through expressive arts therapy.

Way, John B. *Treating Depression.* Hunter College, 1991.

This paper covers the epidemiology, diagnosis and definition of depression. Attention is paid to those who respond poorly to treatment, as well as the major studies showing successful treatment. A review is given of the use of antidepressant drugs, electroshock, and other medical treatments. The major (cognitive/behavioral and interpersonal) psychotherapies are reviewed as well as the evidence that exercise, relaxation, and meditation are valuable. The relevance of the perspectives of bioenergetics, T'ai Chi and dance/movement therapy are considered. The treatment of professional burnout is presented. In conclusion proposals are given of how to best understand depression's occurrence, diagnosis, and treatment as well as suggesting further research that is needed, and programmatic proposals for group programs concerning both treatment and the staff that deliver treatment.

Wegrich, Eileen A. *The Use of Dance/Movement Therapy With an Attention Deficit Hyperactive Disorder Child*. University of California, Los Angeles, 1993.

This thesis presents a clinical case study on a child diagnosed as Attention Deficit Hyperactive Disorder (ADHD). It includes a review of the literature, clinical observations and a means of monitoring the child's psychological and behavioral states following dance/movement therapy. A discussion of clinical impressions on the child's progress and an analysis of the data obtained by the study are presented.

The author's approach to the problem incorporates therapeutic interventions that maypromote an awareness of emotional release, self-control, and empowerment by means of progressive muscle relaxation (PMR) techniques, body awareness, covert rehearsal, play enactments, and dance/ movement therapy activities.

Wegrzyn, Ilana. *Dance Movement Therapy: Case Study of a Latency Age Female with Non-Disclosure of Sexual Abuse*. Laban Centre for Movement and Dance, 1993.

Welssman, Tamar Zur. *Dancing in War Time*. Lesley College Graduate School, 1993.

The Gulf War in 1991 posed for Israel the first experience of the threat of a chemical attack against the civilian population. For six weeks, ground-to-ground missiles were aimed directly at areas of dense population, threatening Israel with death and destruction. Israeli residents experienced eighteen missile attacks and five false alarms. Thirty-nine Scud missiles were fired at Israel. One Scud missile exploded in the center of Hatikva neighborhood and caused severe destruction to homes and public buildings, including the Beit Dani Community Center. The threat to life, loss of property and the destruction imposed a continuing state of stress. As director of the Beit-Dani Dance Group, the author felt deeply involved with the local citizens and especially with the girls of her dance group. She maintained close contact with the girls by visiting them in their homes and at the hotels to which they were evacuated. Ten days after the missile fell, they started dancing again.

This paper describes the history of the dance group of Beit-Dani in war time. The historical background of the concept of stress and theories of stress and anxiety arereviewed. The wartime situation and its influence on individuals, methods of coping, and handling stressful situations are reviewd as well as dance therapy theory and the beneficial therapeutic aspects of dance in times of stress.

Wert, Heidi Beth. *A Mennonite Perspective: Can It Enhance the Helping Professional's Practice?* Hunter College, 1992.

This paper discusses the universal and particularistic aspects of the Mennonite faith. Implications for applying Mennonite philosophy during practice in the social work/dance therapy field is discussed. This paper advocates that helping professionals explore their roots to enhance their practice. Biblical references to social welfare and dance are listed in appendix form and a human sexuality resource list is included.

Westwood, Gregg. *Dance/Movement Therapy: A Vital Adjunctive Treatment for Persons Living with AIDS: A Catalyst for Change*. Naropa Institute, 1995.

A research study was conducted on the effects that dance/movement therapy may have on the physical, psychological, and social functioning of persons living with AIDS. Four men participated in a dance/movement therapy group for fifteen weeks, culminating in a performance. They were administered a quality of life assessment before and after the process, and participated in a qualitative interview process.

The results speculate that dance/movement therapy can be a catalyst for physical, psychological and social change for persons living with AIDS. A video of the performance is submitted along with the thesis.

Wilkinson, Amanda. *The Use of Inner Awareness and the Process of Self-Transformation in Lines Ballet Company Dancers: The Relationship to Dance/Movement Therapy Practice.* University of California, Los Angeles, 1995. (SP)

Williams, Amy. *Dance/Movement Therapy and Drama Therapy As Co-Modalities with an Adolescent Population.* Antioch/New England Graduate School. 1994.

The purpose of this study is to investigate the assumption that dance/movement therapy and drama therapy are effective co-modalities for an adolescent population. Specific movement interventions, as well as dramatic choices, are documented and examined with a group of adolescents. The change in emotional states and movement role preference is measured by portions of the Kestenberg Movement Profile (KMP) and Piers-Harris Children's Self Concept Scale. Movement preferences, role and thematic preferences, and the relationship between the two are explored. Three females and three males, ages 14-18, are assessed via video footage at the beginning and at the end of at least a four month period involvement with an improvisational, issue-oriented, audience-interactive, theater training troupe, called ACTING OUT. This footage was notated by the author using tension-flow portions of the KMP. The Piers-Harris Children's Self Concept Scale was administered at the same intervals as the movement profiles. Recommendations are made for treatment strategies and goal setting in a group such as this and ideas for further research are offered.

Williams, Sara J. *Choreography of The Parts of The Self: A Heuristic Study in Wholeness.* Antioch/New England Graduate School, 1995.

The process of the choreography of the parts of the self is presented through heuristic research. Heuristic research is made up of three phases; immersion, acquisition, and realization. Working within heuristic methodology, parts of the self were explored through creative and expressive arts. The data collected in each phase were personal journal writings, art work, conversations on tape, reflections on the creative process, and choreography, all of which brought me to a deeper understanding of my self. The emergence and subsequent integration of parts of the self within heuristic research phases allowed for the exploration of foreign, inner landscapes.

Williams, Susan R. *Seasons of Darkness And Light: The Earth as a Guide For The Dance/Movement Therapist-in-Training.* Antioch/New England Graduate School, 1993.

This thesis explores the connection between the self-creating ability of the Earth and the experiences of creative chaos, symbolic death, and rebirth that the dance/movement therapist may undergo in preparing to work effectively in the mental health field. A review of literature on the creative process and psychotherapeutic training is discussed. A workshop with rain forest advocate, John Seed, was integrated into this study as part of the research on the Earth and our human connections to the natural world. Included is a chapter on the Earth-loving shaman, whose call to the healing profession necessitates a journey through the abyss. A survey, distributed to first, second, and third year students of Antioch's program in Dance/Movement Therapy, was used to determine the extent to which death/rebirth themes have played a role in the training process. This thesis suggests that the dance/movement therapist-in-training may experience significant challenges to his/her sense of identity and that the Earth can be viewed as an omnipresent, trustworthy, and effective guide through the creative process of death of the old self and rebirth of the new.

Winborne, Valerie A. *Dance/Movement Therapy as a Treatment Modality in Healing Depression in Women*. New York University, 1991.

This study presents the collaboration of a traditional therapist and a dance/movement therapist regarding a case of a 33 year old Chinese woman suffering from clinical depression. The author reviews: the creative arts therapies as the missing links in treating mental illness, statistics on depression, and women and mental health. She comes to the conclusion that traditional methods of treatment like psychiatry and psychology have created inefficient, costly and time consuming practices. Dance/movement therapy was implemented twice a week to complement therapy. It was expected that it would have a positive impact on the patient's treatment. The patient showed marked improvement in verbal therapy and many other areas. Discussed are the implications for dance/movement therapy to enhance traditional methods of therapy.

Wisel, Lisa. *Profile of Nonverbal Indicators of Aggression: A Dance Therapist's Perspective*. Hunter College, 1991.

This paper focuses on aggressive behavior and the specific characteristics of the psychiatric patient in the hospital setting. Consideration was given to various aspects of aggression, definitions, scales and theoretical frameworks. Assessment, treatment planning and management for the assaultive patient are discussed.

The Long Beach Memorial Hospital's aggressive profile, which was developed in collaboration with a multi-disciplinary treatment team is presented. It was designed to provide staff with cues to potentially violent behavior. Terms are defined and methods for clinical use of the profile are covered.

Specific implications for dance/movement therapy are explored. A list of movements during moments of increased aggressive tension is included along with dance/movement therapy interventions.

Wissinger, Anne-Louise. *Dance/Movement Therapy and Children with Learning Disabilities: A Perceptual Motor Approach*. Hunter College, 1994.

The focus of this thesis is on using dance/movement therapy, in combination with perceptual motor approaches to treat children with learning disabilities. Children with learning disabilities are a heterogenous group, with a spectrum of characteristics. These children have at least average learning potential, but have some problems that interfere with normal learning. There are a variety of theories and approaches in dealing with LD children. Little evidence supports the superiority of one approach over another. Perceptual-motor therapy and dance/movement therapy share some common goals and philosophies and are presented herein as effective interventions for children with LD. These theories lend to each other different facets for approaching and treating LD in a diverse and multifaceted manner.

Wittner, Lisa Metill. *Why Dance? Individual Expression and Community Building Through Dance*. Naropa Institute, 1996.

This thesis explores the healing potential of dance. It is suggested that in African-derived cultures dance is an integral part of the culture, filling important needs of people in the society. The ways in which dance provides an opportunity for individual expression and for community building is discussed. A comparison is made in relation to the role of dance in contemporary Euro-American society. It is proposed that dance does not play a central role in this culture and that instead other disciplines have emerged to fill many of the same needs that dance fulfills in traditional cultures. The field of dance therapy is explored as one such practice.

The review of literature contains information on African, Brazilian, Haitian and Cuban cultures, on the role of dance in these cultures, and on dance therapy in the United States. The focus is on the similar role that African dance and dance therapy have in simultaneously supporting individual expression and community. The discussion section explores differences between African and Euro-American cultures and the ways in which dance therapy resurrects an ancient healing art. The research section is comprised of interviews with dance teachers from Senegal, Brazil, Haiti, and the United States and dance therapists from different parts of the United States.

Witzer, Barbara Raymer. *Dance/Movement Therapy With Alcohol and Substance Abuse Patents: Moving Through Resistance.* University of California, Los Angeles, 1992.

The purpose of this thesis is to explore how dance/movement therapy (DMT) can be an effective modality to overcome resistance in alcohol and substance abuse (ASA) patients who are participating in a 28-day alcohol and substance abuse program. The concept of addiction is reviewed and the characteristics of the alcoholic and substance abuser is examined. The author provides a review of the clinical concept of resistance, discusses factors that lead to resistance, explores resistance as displayed through somatic defenses, and presents specific techniques which this writer found useful in DMT sessions with alcohol and substance abusers.

Resistance, for the purpose of this thesis, is defined as "client opposition to change" (Tilley, 1984, p. 14). When resistant, the ASA patent often demonstrates maladaptive somatic defenses. These defenses frequently block the ASA patient's ability to make healthy choices and changes in life. The author focused primarily on the resistance and somatic defenses of the ASA patient within the dance/movement therapy sessions. The following seven techniques were found beneficial to lessen resistance and work through somatic defenses: body awareness, relaxation techniques, body focusing, body and movement metaphors, creating personal space, imagery, and the observation of other patients. These are described and clinical examples which examine the impact of these techniques are given. The thesis concludes with a summary of the implications and value of using DMT in a 28-day alcohol and substance abuse program.

Wolf, Brigitte. *Movement Preferences and Interactions of Emotionally and Behaviorally Disturbed Adolescents in Relation to Moral Development and Perspective-Taking Skills.* Naropa Institute, 1994.

This study looks at possible movement factors of interpersonal interactions and of movement preferences that relate to moral developmental stages and to perspective-taking skills. Since a relationship has been found by other authors between moral development and perspective-taking, it was hypothesized that a relationship to physical perspective-taking such as in mirroring can be found as well. Furthermore, moral developmental stages and/or perspective-taking are visible in movement patterns.

Four male adolescents, three from a program for emotionally and behaviorally disturbed adolescents and one normal boy, were observed as case studies. They were given a Kohlberg questionnaire and a perspective-taking task to determine their developmental stage. In addition they were asked to perform two mirroring exercises and a role play with a partner. The activities were videotaped and later analyzed for the participants degree of matching each other and their time spent on acting and distracting. The subjects were also observed according to a movement scale.

The results are not definite, but some possible relations could be seen, such as a relation of sagittal body attitude to pre-conventional, horizontal stress to conventional and vertical attitude to post-conventional levels of moral development. A list of the movement factors in interpersonal interactions and of movement preferences that seem to relate to moral developmental stages and to perspective-taking skills are given. This may help focus further research in this area.

Wolpert, Joyce B. *Self Esteem: Dance/Movement Therapy and Movement Observation with Emotionally Disturbed Adolescent Boys.* Goucher College, 1992.

This study explores the relationship between dance/movement therapy and self esteem in emotionally disturbed adolescent boys. Literature is reviewed from the areas of normal adolescent development, emotional disturbance in adolescents, self esteem, movement observation and dance/movement therapy process, methods and techniques. The topic is developed by creating a Movement Observation Scale with nineteen Laban Effort-Shape parameters equated with self esteem, as gathered from previous studies in the field. The hypothesis is that dance/movement therapy works to increase the number of observable movement behaviors equated with self esteem in emotionally disturbed adolescent boys. The author conducted a series of ten individual sessions for each of four boys from a residential treatment center for emotionally disturbed adolescents. The first, fifth and tenth sessions were videotaped and clinical notes were kept on the therapy process. A Certified Movement Analyst (CMA) and Registered Dance Therapist (ADTR), reviewed the tapes and rated the movement behaviors according to the scale. Results, presented both in chart and case narrative form, indicated that dance/movement therapy was a moderately effective tool in increasing movement behaviors equated with self esteem. Each of the boys demonstrated progress along some of the parameters with the greatest progress being made in the use of Weight Effort, Weight and Space Inner Attitude, and the use of Shape. These results were interpreted to mean that the subjects were able to demonstrate more Weight Effort when their affect levels (particularly excitement or anger) increased, and in the case of Weight and Space, and Shape when doing certain tasks and games that helped them display their mastery and thus increased their sense of self. Future research is suggested along the lines of creation of a valid movement observation scale for this population, refinement of scale parameters and development of a more accurate measurement to discriminate among adolescent subgroups.

Woods, Lora. *The Use of Dance/Movement Therapy with Hospital Personnel.* University of California, Los Angeles, 1993.(SP)

Yeager, Lindsey. *A Movement Therapy Based Treatment Program for Negative Body Image in Adolescent Females.* University of California, Los Angeles, 1996.

A treatment model for negative body image and its associated features of lowered self-esteem and depression in adolescent females is proposed, implemented and tested for its effectiveness in the form of two "process-outcome" pilot studies. The model of treatment follows a "movement therapy based psychoeducational prevention and intervention" approach designed by the author. Its effectiveness is tested with two different populations; a nonclinical population of four adolescent females in a preventative setting (YWCA), and a clinical population of four adolescent females in an intervention facility (residential treatment). Both quantitative and qualitative measures were collected prior to and following the intervention. Quantitative measures include the Multidimensional Body-Self Relations Questionnaire (Cash, Winstead & Janda, 1986), the Rosenberg Self-Esteem Scale (Rosenberg, 1965), and the Children's Depression Inventory. Qualitative measures include participants' journal entries and comments during the program. The clinical pilot study was compared against a control group. A strong pattern of responses emerged in favor of effectiveness of the treatment model for negative body image and depression. Body image scores improved in seventy-five percent of all participants and depression scores decreased in sixty-three percent of all participants. Qualitative measures indicated increased self expression and improved self-concept as well among all participants. The outcome of these two pilot studies suggests a strong need for a treatment program for negative body image among both nonclinical and clinical female adolescent populations.

Yuval, Merav. *Dance Movement Therapy With Pediatric Oncology Patients.* Hunter College, 1995.

This is an explorative investigation of the use of dance movement therapy in a pediatric oncology setting. The premise of this study is that dance movement therapy provides children with leukemia a unique form of expression which may facilitate a significant psychological, emotional and cognitive change and enhance their sense of well-being. Literature of childrens' cancer, its treatment and its psychological effect is reviewed as well as childrens' developmental theories. A variety of current psychological interventions in pediatric oncology and theories regarding dance movement therapy are presented. A series of clinical group dance movement therapy sessions with children at ages 8 and 9 years, diagnosed with leukemia, are presented in order to illustrate the use of dance movement therapy in a pediatric oncology setting.

Zachos, Dimitrios. *An Exploration from a Structural Point of View of the Use of the Greek Traditional Form of Dance in a Dance Movement Therapy Group of Greek Schizophrenic Patients.* Laban Centre for Movement and Dance, 1995.

Zenstein, Cherie I. *A Theoretical Rationale for Using Reminiscence in Dance/Movement with Depressed Elderly People.* Allegheny University of the Health Sciences (formerly Hahnemann University), 1994.

This thesis proposes a theoretical rationale for using reminiscence in dance/movement therapy with depressed elderly people. Elderly patients experience a wide variety of emotional responses to a pattern of constant losses and readjustments in the last cycle of their lives. Psychotherapy is believed to be effective for this population in coping with their losses and developing a support system. Dance/movement therapy is a psychotherapeutic approach which incorporates the cognitive and verbal with the emotional and the non-verbal. Reminiscence in dance/movement therapy may be a powerful approach where the elderly can identify their feelings and find some resolution with their past, preparing them for death. When performing a movement that reminds them of past mastery experiences, depressed elderly people often appear alert and organized. This thesis concludes that reminiscing in group dance/movement therapy sessions results in interaction which can help the socially depressed and isolated. With consideration of the areas in the brain responsible for recall of memory through movement, a theoretical rationale is developed and discussed regarding reminiscence in dance/movement therapy with depressed elderly people.

Zern, Catherine G. *Ego Mechanisms of Defense and Body Movement in the Borderline Personality.* Goucher College, 1994.

The purpose of this study is to examine the relationship between body movement patterns and ego mechanisms of defense, exploring whether such a relationship exists, and if so, how this relationship manifests itself. The question is applied specifically to the borderline personality disordered population. Theory and definitions explicating ego defense mechanisms are presented. The clinical portrait of the borderline personality, including character traits, characteristic object relations, and intrapsychic conflicts is provided for the reader. The concepts and applications of Labanalysis are described, and their relevance to the thesis question discussed.

A total of eleven psychotherapists were interviewed individually. In the first group, psychotherapists elaborated on their clinical experiences with borderline individuals and their observations regarding associated ego defenses. The second group, comprised of psychotherapists with certification in movement analysis, presented their observations on both movement characteristics and ego defenses seen in this population. Interview findings are summarized in narrative form and examined in the context of the literature review. The literature and the results of the interviews suggest that there is a relationship between individual body movement patterns and the borderline individual. Effort and collapse, fluidity of presentation, a broader repertoire of movement than utilized, lack of shaping, difficulty using "authentic" movement, and lack of containment on a body level are characteristics that appear to be associated with the borderline personality. The relationship, however, between specific ego defenses and body movement in this population is less clear. The author suggests that numerous studies in this area must be accomplished before any definitive statements can be made. The need for empirical research is emphasized and possibilities for future research proposed.

Zimbelmann, Christine. *Grief and Loss: Rebirth Through Dance Therapy.* Hunter College, 1991.

Loss and grief are universal human experiences and as such must be addressed by the dance therapist. In this thesis the literature on loss, grief and bereavement is explored. The focus of this exploration is on the symptoms of grief, the stages of grieving, the funeral ritual (it's purposes and characteristics in Western vs. non-Western cultures), and on the various treatment modalities used with the bereaved. Because of the de-ritualization and emphasis on suppression of emotion in Western culture today, there are many people who have been unable to find an appropriate outlet for the feelings of sadness, guilt and anger which typically accompany a loss. The discussion is a theoretical look at how dance therapy, due to it's basic principles, might be instrumental in enabling those who have not grieved or are "stuck" in their grief, to express their feelings and to work through their grief. A comparison is made between the funeral ritual and the dance therapy session. Based on this comparison one might conclude that due to its inherent principles, dance therapy may ultimately be instrumental in guiding us through the inevitable losses in our lives.

Ziv, Anat. *Dance and Movement Therapy with Pregnant Women: A Multicultural Study.* California State University, Hayward, 1993.

The purpose of this thesis was to examine the efficacy of dance/movement therapy in working with pregnant women living away from their home countries. Dance/movement therapy interventions were used to establish a support group and to ease the difficulties of pregnancy: to decrease anxiety level, increase self-awareness, release body tension, build stronger self-esteem and increase trust in the body's ability to cope with stressful situations. The connection between object-relations and pregnancy perception and the correlation between culture and pregnancy and its expression in movment, were observed during the sessions. Laban movement analysis helped the investigator to observe and analyze the women's movement.

Index

Index

Abuse
Pupello, P.A.

Addictions
Egido, E.M.; Goehring, C.G.: Morton, P.; Steinberger, D.; Watson, L.D.; Witzer, B.R.

Adolescence
Abrahamson, G.; Audette, C.; Binette, L.; Booth, H.; Briski, M.K.; Chapek, K.; Connell, J.; Cooper, A.C.; Correa, M.; Danner, J.; Dillman, D.S.; Farr, M.; Fowler, B.B.; Fucius, Y.; Goldschlag-Teich, M.; Haney, T.; Higgins, S.; Hurst, S.M.; Lewis, G.E.; Morningstar, D.; Nixon, A.; Ojala, E.; Parasuram, K.; Peterson, K.M.; Radcliffe, N.; Rupp, A.; Scholefield, J.; Selzman, L.J.; Trott, M.; Vella, G.E.; Venable, E.I.; Watkins, A.R.; Williams, A.; Wolf, B.; Wolpert, J.B.; Yeager, L.;

Affective Expression
Burt, J.W; DeLeon F.; Hudak, K.M.; McGuire, l.; Nadvornik, K.A.

Affect Theory
Maciel,D.

African-American
Alexander, P.; Davis, C.V.; Farr, M.; Fountaine, L.H.; Harmon, N.K.; Lowery, T.; Sutton-Randolph, C.

Aggression
Connell, J.; Nixon, A.; Wisel,L.

AIDS
Coburn, L.; Comer, M.E.; Foglietti, R.; Hartstein, J.L.; Hiller, C.A.; Westwood, G.

Alexithymia
Rumrill, M.R.

Alzheimer's Disease
Boone, E.A.; Parland, N.M.

Anxieties
Chutroo, B.; Kitt, A.L.; Maxwell, T.A.; Nadvornik, K.A.

Assertiveness
Lowery, T.

Assessments
Anderson, K.R.; Brenner, T.; Cruz, R.F.; Hey, J.; O'Toole, B.; Rieder, A.S.; Tangstad, A.B.

Attention Deficit Hyperactivity Disorder
Burns, C.; Gorscak, K.J.; MacKay, F.K.; Noble, E.A.; Steckert, K.; Wegrich, E.A.

Authentic Movement
Angeloro, V.M.; Bryson, R.C.; Correa, M.; Kohl, M.; Menzam, C.; Parry,, A.; Rothermel, L.

Autism
Azizollahof, J.; Daigle, R.; Davis, A.; Economou, K.; Gonzales, P.S.; Gronlund, E.; Hedson, A.B.; Karash, A.; McGehee, S.; North, C.; Ray, D.; Raynor, R.M.; Rivi, D.; Smith, P.; Stent, D.

Battered Females
Cerami, F.

Behavioral Disorders
Durkin, C.

Body Boundaries
Kasovac, N.; Steckert, K.

Body Image
Angert, G.; Becker, M.G.; Brown, K.; Conwell, C.; Fishbein, T.; Gross, C.; Kwon, E.H.; McFadden, M.; Selzman, L.J.; Yeager, L.

Body Memory
Case, V.

Body-Mind
Berger, M.R.; Burden, K.A.; Foglietti, R.; Ginga, M.; Hallmark, E.; North, C.; Rothermel, L.

Body Therapies
Eaton, B.; Burden, K.A.

Borderline Personality Disorder
Levidi, E.; Perrin, A.M.; Simpson, A.; Thomas, D.; Vella, G.E.; Vorspan, R.; Zern, C.G.

Brain Functions
Smith, P.; Watson, L.D.

Brain and Head Injuries
Connell, D.; Goldman, L.; Guthrie, J.; Lorenz, C.H.; Mettler, T.A.; Morris, C.B.

Breath
Hale, L.S.; Klotzkin, J.

Cardiac Rehabilitation
Hyle, D.

Centering
Schultz, R.

Cerebral Palsy
Parasuram, K.

Chace, Marian
Berger, M.R.; Brandt, K.; Brodersohn, A.; Huber, W.F.

Children
Arcuri, C.B.; Baker, M.F.; Bond, K.E.; Brauninger, I.; Brennan, E.R.; Brenner, T.; Brown, K.; Burns, F.; Clauer, M.; Cowen, H.; Durkin, C.; Errington, A.; Fear, L.; Fishbein, T.; Gellman, L.; Goldsand, R.A.; Gonnella, N.; Gonzalez, C.A.; Gronlund, E.; Hayes, J.S.; Hrushovski, T.; Jackson, S.; Kram, C.D.; Kwon, E.H.; Levin, C.; Mackay, F.K.; Moore, M.; North, C.; Olsen, J.; Omeragic-Mestanagic, G.; Pupello, P.A.; Reed, R.; Sawyer, A.D.; Tsunemine, Y.; Watney, L.; Wegrzyn, I.; Yuval, M.

Chronic Illness
Isecke, M.; Noel, L.G; Yuval, M.

Chronic Mental Illness
Rice, R.

Chronic Pain
Gray, S.; Janco, O.; Sargent, L.; Sheble, M.S.; Schalkwijk-Vanderkruk, M.E.

Circle
Adams, S.L.; Connors, J.; Moroney, T.; Thelen, J.A.

Communication Problems
Schingo, F.

Community
Ashley, J.S.; LeBeaux, C.G.; Leighton, F.E.

Co-Therapy
Hudson, K.A.

Counter-Indications
Bennett, E.

Counter-Transference
Hollander, M.E.; Matias, M.; Omeragic-Mestanagic, G.; Scapini-Burrell, I.; Tsunemine, Y.

Creative Process
Booth, H.; Few, J.B.; Gowen, G.; Kaspi, O.; Miller, B.; Parland, N.M.; Shaban, H.; Williams, S.R.

Cross-Cultural
Adderley, M; Alexander, P.; Arakawa, K.; Benvenuto, J.; Cohen, J.; DeJean, D.; Dripchak, V.; El Guindry, H.; Embers, J.; Jingu, K.; Johns, S.D.; Landau, A.; Minott, D.Y.; Neglia, N.A.; Parra, L.; Prettyman, M.; Thomas, K.A.; Wittner, L.M.; Ziv, A.

Dance
Adderley, M.; Alexander, P.; Ben-Moshe, A.; Binette, L.; Browne, W.R.; Chapek, K.; Connors, J.; El Guindry, H.; Goldschlag-Teich, M.; Johns S.D.; Landau, A.; Leeds, M.; Nemetz, L.D.; Rubenstein, J.; Schmoelz-Schappin, N.; Shaw, B.; Szuszan, M.; Tupa, R.; Weissman, T.Z.; Wilkinson, A.; Wittner, L.M.; Zachos, D.

Dance/Movement Therapy: Career Choice
Boyle, B.; Hallmark, E.; Orth, C.; Stepek, H.L.

Dance/Movement Therapy History
Brandt, K.; Brodersohn, A.; DiPalma, E.M.

Dance/Movement Therapy Process
Hey, J; O'Reilly, E.M.

Dance/Movement Therapy Programs
Arner, J.; Faraone, C.J.; Gary, G.; Moyer-Holmberg, M.; Musacchio, J.; Oglesby, T.K.; Plattner, M.

Dance/Movement Therapy Students
Abrahamsen, S.J.; Arner, J.; Moyer-Holmberg, M.; O'Reilly, E.M.; Plattner, M.; Sheppard, P.E.; Williams, S.R.

Dance/Movement Therapy Theory
Arndt, C.; Berger, M.R.; Coburn, L.; DiNoto, L.M.; DiPalma, E.M.; Jacoby, R.; Kahlen, M.R.; Press, E.; Risher, E.A.; Rozen, L.M.; Scudder, A.T.; Thomas, D.; Torp, C.

Deafness
Comyn, A.; Cooper, A.C.; Simon, J.; Strickler, S.A.

Defense Mechanisms
DeBeer, E.; Sherrill, J.M.; Watson, L.D.; Zern, C.G.

Dementia (also see Elderly)
Hill, H.

Depression
Balish-LaSaine, D.; Briski, M.K.; Clauer, M.; Higgins, S.; Irving, D.; Kinni, E.; Kram, C.D.; Rosenberg, T.; Scholefield, J.; Schwartz, C.; Vella, G.E.; Way, J.B.; Winborne, V.A.; Zenstein, C.I.

Developmentally Delayed: See Mental Retardation

Developmental Stages
Davis, A.; Egido, E.M.; Fishbein, T.; Glenn, M.; Levinbook-Mezamer, M.; Lucier, C.F; Nemetz, L.D.; North, C.; Olsen, J.; Ruth, T.T.; Steinberg, S.; Strickler, S.A.

Down's Syndrome
Bertz, J.M.; Giannone, G.M.; Watney, L.

Drama
Few, J.B.; Wallace, J.; Williams, A.

Dreams
Himmelgreen, C.; Ward, C.D.

Dual Diagnoses
Hayes, L; Matias, M.; Radcliffe, N.; Sussman, S.

Index

Eastern Philosophies
Leighton, F.E.; Risher, E.A.; Rochell, D.M.; Scudder, A.T.; Umiguchi, Y.

Eating Disorders
Abrahamsen, S.J.; Bauer, S.; Fowler, B.B.; Funderburk, J.B.; Goss, H.C.; Hugill, T.; Prud'homme, S.A.; Shahar, T.; Stern, H.

Educational Settings
Chyorny, R.; Leahy, D.

Elderly
Anderson, K.R.; Angert, G.; Boone, E.A.; Crowley, R.; Hill, H.; Irving, D.; Koshland, L.M.; Morrissee, C.M.; Parland, N.M.; Samuels, A.; Trachtenberg, K.G.; Zenstein, C.I.

Emotionally Disturbed Adolescents (see Adolescents)
Green, N.M.; Peterson, K.M.; Wolpert, J.B.

Emotionally Disturbed Children (see Children)
Baker, M.F.; Durkin, C.; Jackson, S.; Levinbook-Mezamer, M.; Millrod, E.T.; Trainor, M.; Visconti, D.M.

Empathy
Fraenkel, D.L.; Goldman-Nevins, K.L.; Rasmussen, T.

Emptiness
Thomas, D.

Encounter Groups
Arner, J.

Energy
Lucas, P.A.; Scudder, A.T.

Evil
Lucas, P.A.

Family
Mesmer, A.C.; Moore, C.A.

Family Therapy
Falk, M.G.; Stone, S.

Fetish
Kwon, E.H.

Gender
Boyle, B.; Hudak, K.M.

Grief
Booth, H.; Isis, K.B.; Mesmer, A.C.; Sussman, S.; Zimbelmann, C.

Group Dance/Movement Therapy
Bradshaw, G.; Cohen, A.E.; Dillman, D.S.; Gonnella, N.; Greene, S.W.; Hayes, L.; Moncrieff, M.; Nagy, I.; Venable,, E.I.; Ward, C.D.

Group Process
Moncrieff, M.

Holistic Health
Keck, A.E.

Homelessness
Phipps, K.M.; Torp, C.

Homosexuality
Comer, M.E.; Larsen, K.E.

Humor
Papastratigaki, M.

Hypnotherapy
Kennedy, J.R.

Imagery
Chenier, K.B.; Shahar, T.; Thorpe, L.B.

Improvisation
Chapek, K.

Intergenerational
Morrissee, C.M.; Rose, S.C.

Infants
Burt, J.W.; Venable, E.T.

Jungian Theory
Brennan, E.R.; Cowen, H.; Fleischer, K.; Goldman, D.R.; Gowen, G.; Parry, A.

Kestenberg Movement Profile
Atley, S.H.; Berger, K.; Binette, L.; Brenner, T.; Burden, K.A.; Curtin, P.; Daigle, R.; Fischbach, M.; Goldstein, L.I.; Hurst, S.M.; Lemon, J.; Ojala, E.; Stupka-Malloy, A.; Watkins, A.R.; Williams, A.

Kinesthetic Empathy
Berger, M.R.; Goldman-Nevins, K.L.

Learning Disabilities
Goldstein, L.I.; Jackson, S.; Wissinger, A.L.

Mental Retardation
Blatz, A.; Hazama, E.; McClanahan, K.; Moogan, L.; Ojala, E.

Metaphor
Becker, M.G.

Minimal Brain Dysfunction
Hrushovski, T.

Mirroring
Papastratigaki, M.

Mother/Child
Daigle, R.; Lucier, C.F.; Rivi, D.; Venable, E.T.

Movement Observation
Ahroni (Barkai), Y.; Bertz, J.M.; Connolly, K.; De Jesus, M.; Gorscak, K.J.; Guthrie, J.; Moogan, L.; Morningstar, D.; O'Toole, B.; Ray, D.; Wolpert, J.B.

Movement Patterns
Brauninger, I.; Cruz, R.F.; DeArment, M.; Gowen, G.; Hale, L.S.; Har-El Belach, R.; Maskens, K.; Menzam, C.; Moore, C.A.; Rieder, A.S.; Wolf, B.; Zern, C.G.

Multiple Personality Disorder
Arning, J.; Bartko, D.P.; Connolly, K.; DeArment, M.

Multiply Handicapped
Correa, M.

Music
Ben-Dor, K.; Lewis, G.E.; Sutton-Randolph, C.

Myth
Curtin, P.; Goldman, D.R.; Himmelgreen, C.; Szuszan, M.; Vincent, N.B.

Nonverbal Behavior
Burt, J.W.; Cohen, A.E.; Fountaine, L.H.; Fraenkel, D.L.; Ran, F.; Schingo, F.

Object Relations
Burns, C.; Cowen, H.; Davis, A.; Geller, J.; Gronlund, E.; Henry, J.T.; Hrushovski, T.; Kwon, E.H.; Levinbook-Mezamer, M.; Millrod, E.T.

Obsessive Compulsive Disorder
Arakawa, K.; Clarke, M.S.

Oncology
Franken, F.; Moskow, J.; Noel, L.G.; Rider, M.L.; Yuval, M.

Organizational Systems
Brady, S.; Schingo, F.

Osteoarthritis
Angert, G.

Parkinson's Disease
Bunce, J.M.

Performance
Wallace, J.

Personal Growth
Chutroo, B.; Diaz-Salazar, P.; DiNoto, L.M.; Glenn, M.; Majoris, D.; Schmoelz-Schappin, N.; Sheppard, P.E.; Vorspan, R.; Williams, S.J.

Personality Disorders
Federman, D.

Personality Traits
Har-El Belach, R.; Orth, C.; Stepek, H.L.

Physical Illnesses
Bunce, J.M.; Fear, L.; Franken, F.; Frant, P.; Ginga, M.; Moskow, J.; Rider, M.L.

Physical Rehabilitation
Eckhaus, N.S.; Tangstad, A.B.

Play
Brennan, E.R.; Brower, D.; Curtis, S.; Greene, S.W.; Lucier, C.F.; MacArthur, L.; Millrod, E.T.; Tsunemine, Y.

Post Traumatic Stress Disorder
Fischbach, M.; Gonzalez, C.A.; Thurston, C.J.; Tobler, A.C.

Pregnancy
Ziv, A.

Prevention
Keyeski, J.; McFadden, M.A.; Woods, L.

Prisoners
Guffy, J.

Private Practice
Stone, R.

Process Oriented Therapy
Funderburk, J.B.; Leahy, D.

Professional Development
Boyle, B.; Glenski, R.; Hallmark, E.; LeBeaux, C.G.; Nace, F.; Norman, V.; Stone, R.

Professional Status
Dillian, C.E.; Luca, K.

Props
Mackay, F.K.

Psychoeducational Treatment
Azizollahoff, J.; Schalkwijk-Vanderkruk, M.E.; Yeager, L.

Psychosocial Rehabilitation
Chessman, P.; Rice, R.

Psychosomatic Disorder
Isecke, M.

Public School Setting
Bram, D.L.; Chyorny, R.; Danner, J.; Davies, M.I.; Durkin, C.; Green, N.M.; LeBeaux, C.G.; Trainor, M.

Publication
Norman, V.; Schmoelz-Schappin, N.

Reference Materials
Fledderjohn, H.; Rikita, C.; Sewickley, J.

Relational Model
Sargent, L.; Trinkley, M.; Watkins, A.R.

Relationships
Hayes, J.S.; Hurst, S.M.; Romer, M.B.; Tupa, R.

Religion
Wert, H.B.

Reminiscence
Zenstein, C.I.

Research
Rozen, L.M.; Bond, K.E.

Resistance
Champlin, K.; Witzer, B.R.

Rhythm
Dolin, J.; McGehee, S.; Moroney, T.; Nagy, I.; Pereira-Stubbs, F.

Rituals
Bryson, R.C.; Gaudreau, R.; Perea, P.E.

Schizophrenia
Betjemann, T.; Blaha, J.; Brown, P.J.; Howard, K.; Moroney, T.; Papillon, S.A.; Ray, D.; Steinberg, S.; Thelen, J.

Self-Concept
Blatz, A.; Brown, K.; Cerami, F.; Dolin, J.E.; Levidi, E.; Wallace, J.

Self-Esteem
DeBeer, E.; Khodl, N.A.; Ran, F.; Trott, M.; Wolpert, J.

Sensory Impairment
Bond, K.E.

Sexual Abuse
Bradshaw, G.; Brenner, T.; Farone, D.; Fischbach, M.; Goldsand, R.A.; Kinsey, V.; Lemessurier, C.; Moore, M.; Reed, R.S.; Rochell, D.M.; Schindler, S.; Wegrzyn, T.

Sexual Agression
Brennan, E.R.; Morningstar, D.; Turner, T.N.

Shamanism
Quealy, M.L.

Shame
Jasperse, K.

Short Term Dance/Movement Therapy
Peterson, K.M.; Schwartz, C.

Social Interaction
Cornwall, R.P.; Giannone, G.M.; Koshland, L.M.; Morrissee, C.M.; Samuels, A.; Turkenitz, T.

Social Work
Cohen, A.E.; Rasmussen, T.; Rosenberg, T.

Space
Phipps, K.M.

Special Education
Bram, D.L.; Cornwall, R.P.; Green, N.M.; Minott, D.Y.; Trainor, M.

Spirituality
Ashley, J.S.; Browne, W.R.; Curtin, P.; Efferding, M.J.; Embers, J.; Lipschutz, R.; Miller, B.

Storytelling
Turner, T.N.; Vincent, N.B.

Stress Management
Hyle, D.; Masters, K.; Russell, M.; Weissman, T.Z.

Supervision
Neriya, P.P.

Symbolism
Adams, S.L.; Greenberg, W.; Moncrieff, M.; Nagy, I.; Perea, P.E.

Tension
Umiguchi, Y.

Termination
Kram, C.D.

Therapist's Role
Angeloro, V.M.; Berman, J.; Chutroo, B.; Glenn, M.; Kitt, A.L.; Majoris, D.; Nadvornik, K.A.; Romer, M.B.; Schultz, R.; Vorspan, R.

Torture
Callaghan, K.

Touch
Greenberg, R.; Henson, K. B.H.; Nieman, M.S.; Reed, R.S.

Transference
Omeragic-Mestanagic, G.; Parra, L.

Verbalization
Baker, M.F.; Ben-Ami, R.; Borenstein-Saks, M.; Burt, J.W.; Fraenkel, D.L; Greenberg, R.

Verbal Psychotherapy
Kohl, M.; Maxwell, T.A.; Tobler, A.C.

Video Use
Hill, H.

Vietnam Veterans
Tobler, A.C.

Water Therapy
Blaha, J.; Janco, O.; Parr, S.

Women
Balish-LaSaine, D.; Gaudreau, R.; Khodl, N.A.; Lowery, T.; Moorman, L.; Musacchio, J.; Phipps, K.M.; Scarth, S.; Thomas, D.; Trinkley, M.L.; Winborne, V.A.; Ziv, A.

Procedures For Obtaining Dissertations, Theses and Special Projects

The following is a list of the locations where the complete works covered in this volume are housed, as well as information about how these may be obtained. Listed are the institutions which have a dance/movement therapy program or have had such a program within the years 1991-1996.

There are several listed abstracts which were completed in institutions without a program. The reader is advised to contact the reference librarian of the school at which it was written. In some cases, it may be possible to contact the author directly. A membership directory is maintained by the American Dance Therapy Association which may be of assistance in contacting authors. In the case of the special projects abstracted, it will be necessary to contact the author directly.

Doctoral dissertations including those from universities outside the United States are available through the University Microfilms International which is listed below.

American Dance Therapy Association
2000 Century Plaza, Suite 108
10632 Little Patuxent Parkway
Columbia, MD 21044
410-997-4040
410-997-4048 - fax
e-mail: info@ADTA.org

Allegheny University of the Health Sciences
(formerly Hahnemann University)
Allegheny/Hahnemann Library
245 N. 15th St., Mailstop 449
Philadelphia, PA 19102
215-762-7630
Use in library? Yes.
Interlibrary loan? Photocopy for a fee.

Antioch New England Graduate School Library
40 Avon
Keene, NH 03431
603-357-3122 x274
Use in Library? Yes.
Interlibrary loan? Yes.

California State University at Hayward
Not available through library. Contact individual authors through membership list.

Columbia College
600 S, Michigan Avenue
Chicago, IL 60605
312-663-1600 x753
e-mail: library@mail.colum.edu
Use in library? Yes.
Interlibrary loan? No.

Goucher College
1021 Dulaney Valley Road
Towson, MD 21204-2794
410-337-6361.
Use in library? Yes.
Interlibrary loan? Yes.

Hunter College Health Professions Library
425 E. 25th Street
New York, NY 10010
212-481-5117
Use in library? Yes
Interlibrary loan? No

Laban Centre for Movement and Dance
Laurie Grove, New Cross, London SE14 6NH
England
44-181-692-4070 x32
44-181-694-8749 - fax
e-mail: info@laban.co.uk

Lesley College
Graduate School of Arts and Social Sciences
29 Everett Street
Cambridge, MA 02138-2790
Theses are housed in the Dept. of Expressive Therapies
617-349-8437
Use in dept.? Yes.
Photocopy? Yes, for a fee.

Naropa Institute
2130 Arapahoe Avenue
Boulder, CO 80302
303-444-0202 x3507
e-mail: ed@naropa.edu
Use in library? Yes.
Interlibrary loan? Yes.

New York University
Dance Education Program
Dept. of Music and Performing Arts Professions
School of Education
35 W. 4th Street
New York, NY 10012
212-998-5400
e-mail: bergermi@is.nyu.edu
Program director will help interested persons contact authors.

University of California at Los Angeles
410 Hilgard Avenue
Los Angeles, CA 90024
310-825-1323
Use in library? Yes.
Interlibrary loan? Yes.

University Microfilms International
(for dissertations only)
300 N. Zeeb Rd.
Ann Arbor, MI 48106
313-761-4700 or
800-521-3042
This is a service to purchase dissertation reference information and complete dissertations.

Corrections

Should you wish to submit corrections to this volume, please send the following:
- Information as it appears in Volume 2: Name, title, school and year.
- Corrected information.

If your thesis or dissertation was written between 1991-1996 and was not included in this Volume 2, please send the following information:
- Name as it appears on the project.
- Title, school and year submitted.
- Copy of abstract (no chapters).

Include your name, address and phone/email/fax.

Return information to:
Marian Chace Foundation
American Dance Therapy Association
2000 Century Plaza
Suite 108
10632 Little Patuxent Parkway
Columbia, Maryland 21044-3263